Infant and Early Childhood Neuropsychology

Clinical Child Psychology Library

Series Editors: Michael C. Roberts and Annette M. La Greca

ANXIETY AND PHOBIC DISORDERS
A Pragmatic Approach
Wendy K. Silverman and William M. Kurtines

AUTISM
Understanding the Disorder
Gary B. Mesibov, Lynn W. Adams, and Laura G. Klinger

INFANT AND EARLY CHILDHOOD NEUROPSYCHOLOGY
Glen P. Aylward

MANAGING MANAGED CARE
Michael C. Roberts and Linda K. Hurley

PARENT–CHILD INTERACTION THERAPY
Toni L. Hembree-Kigin and Cheryl Bodiford McNeil

SEXUALITY
A Developmental Approach to Problems
Betty N. Gordon and Carolyn S. Schroeder

A Continuation Order Plan is available for this series. A continuation order will bring delivery of each new volume immediately upon publication. Volumes are billed only upon actual shipment. For further information please contact the publisher.

Infant and Early Childhood Neuropsychology

Glen P. Aylward
Southern Illinois University School of Medicine
Springfield, Illinois

Plenum Press • New York and London

Library of Congress Cataloging-in-Publication Data

Aylward, Glen P.
    Infant and early childhood neuropsychology / Glen P. Aylward.
        p.   cm. -- (Clinical child psychology library)
    Includes bibliographical references and index.
    ISBN 0-306-45672-9 (hardcover). -- ISBN 0-306-45673-7 (pbk.)
    1. Pediatric neuropsychology. 2. Infants--Physiology.   I. Title.
II. Series.
    RJ486.5.A95 1997
    618.92'8--dc21   97-30571
                                                               CIP

ISBN 0-306-45672-9 (Hardbound)
ISBN 0-306-45673-7 (Paperback)

© 1997 Plenum Press, New York
A Division of Plenum Publishing Corporation
233 Spring Street, New York, N. Y. 10013

http://www.plenum.com

10 9 8 7 6 5 4 3 2 1

Printed in the United States of America

To Deborah, Shawn, Megan, Brandon, and Mason for their
support and understanding in this endeavor,
love and thanks.

Preface

Clinicians and researchers have become increasingly involved in the neuropsychological assessment of infants and young children. This is related in part to the increasing numbers of infants who now survive insults to the central nervous system and proceed to develop sequelae such as major disabilities (severe mental retardation, cerebral palsy, epilepsy, and sensory impairments) as well as high-prevalence/low-severity dysfunctions (learning, attention, and behavior problems).

Writing this book has provided me with the opportunity to better define and bring together the type of work that I have done over the last 20 years, an area that I call *infant and early childhood neuropsychology*. The discipline is emerging and currently lacks clear definition. Basically, it involves assessment of brain–behavior relationships in the context of developmental change and maturation.

Although there are several good texts on child neuropsychology, this is not the case with infant and early childhood neuropsychology. This reflects in part the fact that the latter is a hybrid and involves neurology, developmental psychology, occupational and physical therapy, and pediatric/child clinical psychology. In this book, I attempt to define the field, describe what is involved in the practice of early developmental neuropsychology, and provide suggestions for further development of the subspecialty.

Because an appreciation of "normal" development is necessary to identify "abnormal" function, description of central nervous system development is provided, followed by conditions indicating how development can be disrupted. Perhaps more unique is the emphasis on assessment and the many conceptual and pragmatic factors that can affect evaluation results. In this subspecialty, clinical practice is not limited to "routine" psychological tests, but also draws from the disciplines mentioned earlier. The interpretive mind-set also differs from other testing situations.

I am indebted to my many mentors in psychology and medicine who over the years have shared their knowledge and patience. I hope this text reflects well on their teachings. I thank the infants and children whom I have evaluated over the last two decades, some of whom through their misfortunes hopefully have allowed us to develop better means of assessment that can somehow positively affect the futures of other children. I am also grateful to the series editors, Michael C. Roberts and Annette La Greca, for their invitation to write the book and their helpful editorial suggestions, and to my editor at Plenum, Mariclaire Cloutier, who "persuasively" kept the publishing process on track. A special thanks is extended to Michelle Macias for her editorial efforts and making sure the medically related information contained herein was accurate.

I hope this book will serve as an initial step for the further development and refinement of the field of infant and early childhood neuropsychology.

GLEN P. AYLWARD

Contents

Infant and Early Childhood
Neuropsychology

What Is Infant and Early Childhood Neuropsychology?

Over the last several decades clinicians and researchers have experienced increased involvement in neurobehavioral assessment of infants and young children. The boundaries between neurology, developmental psychology, occupational/physical therapy, and pediatric/child clinical psychology are not clearly defined; however, it appears that all of these areas offer unique aspects to the neurodevelopmental/neuropsychological evaluation of infants and young children. The resultant hybrid combination of these disciplines could best be termed *infant and early childhood neuropsychology.*

Several years ago, this author stated that neuropsychological assessment of infants and young children was a fledgling area, and this status persists (Aylward, 1988, 1994). The resulting term *early developmental neuropsychology* was defined as "the assessment of brain–behavior relationships in the context of developmental change and maturation" (Aylward, 1988, p. 226). Such assessment is unique, because it occurs against a backdrop of qualitative and quantitative developmental, behavioral, and structural changes, with the velocity of change being greater during this period than any other. The rapidly expanding behavioral repertoire of the infant and young child, and the corresponding divergence of cognitive, motor and neurological functions pose distinct assessment challenges. Moreover, infant and early childhood neuropsychology is an interpretive orientation or mind-set; it involves quantification of qualitative information. More specifically, in many instances the same tests used in other disciplines may be employed, but interpretation of data and the conceptual bases might differ.

TIMELINESS OF THE SUBSPECIALTY

A primary reason for the heightened interest in infant and early childhood neuropsychology is the increasing numbers of infants who now survive some type of insult to the central nervous system (CNS). For example, in premature infants, the limit of viability now is approximately 500 g and 23–24 weeks gestational age (Allen, Donohue, & Dusman, 1993). In addition to preterm birth, such CNS insults include prenatal drug exposure, intrauterine growth retardation, seizures, intraventricular hemorrhage, hydrocephalus, perinatal asphyxia, or hypoxic-ischemic encephalopathy. Along these lines, Risser and Edgell (1988) provided a useful list of examples of possible etiological agents, resultant neural abnormalities, and subsequent neuropsychological findings (see Table 1.1). For example, a genetic disorder might result in a neural abnormality such as microcephaly. The neuropsychological consequence would be mental retardation. The major point is that different etiologies can produce varying structural abnormalities that, in turn, are manifest in various neuropsychological disorders.

The incidence of major disabilities (severe mental retardation, cerebral palsy, epilepsy, and sensory impairments) in children at biological risk has leveled off at approximately 15%–20%, depending on the type of CNS insult and birth weight. However, the incidence (and subsequent prevalence) of less severe, but nonetheless serious disabilities is increasing. These high-prevalence/low-severity dysfunctions include learning, attention, and behavior problems. For example, in the general population, the prevalence of attention deficit disorders is 100 cases per 1000, and learning disorders, 75/1000; however, the prevalence of mental retardation is 20/1000, cerebral palsy 2/1000, severe hearing impair-

Table 1.1. List of Possible Etiological Agents, Neural Abnormalities, and Neuropsychological Consequences

Etiologic agent	Neural abnormality	Neuropsychological outcome
Genetic	Microcephaly	Mental retardation
Nutritional	Regional agenesis	Learning disability
Traumatic	Migratory defect	Attentional disorder
Infectious	Axon/dendrite damage	Sensory loss
Metabolic	Axon/dendrite damage	Motor deficit
Intoxicant	Synaptic loss	Language deficit
Systemic disease	Synaptic aberrance	Speech deficit
Maternal disease	Tissue infarction	Memory disorder
Anoxic-hypoxic	Tissue ischemia	Emotional alteration
Neoplastic	Hemorrhage	Isolated defects
Environmental deprivation	Demyelination	Developmental delay
Idiopathic	Aberrant cell growth	Normal-range functioning
	Gliosis	
	Diffuse	
	Unidentifiable	

Source: Adapted from Risser & Egell (1988). Used with permission.

ment 1.5/1000, and visual impairment 0.4/1000 (Gortmaker, Walker, Weitzman, & Sobol, 1990).

APPLICATIONS

The major applications for infant and early childhood neuropsychological assessment are: (1) to determine the current neurodevelopmental status of the infant or young child, (2) identification of infants who might benefit from intervention, (3) evaluation of the outcome of innovative medical procedures or other interventions, (4) documentation of change in neurodevelopmental status, and (5) prediction of later levels of functioning (outcome).

The age range for infant and early childhood neuropsychology extends from the neonatal period (first 30 days of life) through infancy, and culminates at the toddler/preschool period (up to and including 5 years). Therefore, even within this circumscribed age range, emphasis on neurological, developmental, and intellectual functions and their relationships evolve, with the importance of each varying, depending on age. For example, in the neonatal period, neurological/neurobehavioral functioning typically is assessed. During infancy, developmental (cognitive and motor) as well as neurodevelopmental (e.g., Bayley Infant Neurodevelopmental Screener [BINS], Aylward, 1995) functions are tapped. From approximately 3 years onwards, actual assessment of "intelligence" and other more circumscribed cognitive functions is possible (e.g., Honzik, 1988). Nonetheless, continuity in functions must be identified, and a conceptual framework that could extend across the entire age range is necessary. This type of assessment differs from many traditional, "developmental" evaluation instruments, because of the decreased emphasis on adaptive behaviors (e.g., self-help skills, socialization), as well as the reliance on underlying, neuropsychological conceptual frameworks. In addition to developmental constructs, evaluation of posture, tone, movement, and reflexes also is involved in early neuropsychological assessment.

Clinicians also must consider the interplay between development, recovery of function, and environmental influences whenever they work with children who have been exposed to potential CNS insult. Abnormal early neuropsychological findings could be related to (1) a maturational delay, (2) neural dysfunction, (3) motor deficits, or (4) the influence of variables external to the infant or young child (e.g., behavioral state, temperament, environmental influences, or test limitations). Conversely, the diversity in outcome after CNS insult and "sparing" of functions could be related to absence of residual damage, neural reorganization, behavioral compensation, the consequences of the damage simply not yet emerging, or some combination of these factors. Obviously, this dynamic matrix, in conjunction with the absence of a traditional "gold standard" and the consequences of early brain injury being less certain, causes the diagnostic process to be more complex than at other ages.

Abnormal neuropsychological findings at this age are frequently termed *deficits, delays, lags,* or *retardation,* essentially bringing up the question whether such findings are indicative of pathology or immaturity. Although "delays" and "lags" are noncategorical "diagnoses" under P.L. 99–457 (Education of the Handicapped Act Amendments, 1986), these euphemistic terms imply that there still may be some type of catch-up or behaviors will become normal over time, once brain development is "completed." In actuality this may not be accurate, as abnormal, early neuropsychological findings may indicate a dysfunction, albeit a reversible one. These problems may be "reversible" because of developmental discontinuity in which structure-to-function relations change; and development does not simply progress in a linear manner in terms of the number of elements and interconnections. Rather, development also is a retrogressive process in that major transitions occur in neural and sensory functions, including elimination (remodeling or cell die-back) of more primitive cell assemblies (see Chapter 3). In fact, Prechtl (1984) suggested that such retrogressive processes (i.e., cell death) are prominent 2 months after birth.

DEFINITIONS

Infant and early childhood neuropsychology is synonymous with *early developmental neuropsychology.* However, it is distinct from *pediatric neuropsychology,* which, although incorporating the concept of medical factors affecting the CNS, includes ages that range from childhood through adolescence. *Child neuropsychology, human developmental neuropsychology,* and *child clinical neuropsychology* are other terms used to distinguish child from adult neuropsychology. However, each is distinct from infant and early childhood neuropsychology, primarily because of the strong developmental/neurodevelopmental orientation in the infant and early childhood area. All of these neuropsychological approaches emphasize the fact that one cannot simply downscale and apply adult neuropsychological techniques to infants and young children; rather the direction needs to move "bottom-up" from the neonatal period upwards.

EARLY CNS DAMAGE

Damage to the developing CNS produces impairments that are both qualitatively and quantitatively different from those found in the case of damage to the adult CNS, which further complicates assessment and prediction in infant and early childhood neuropsychology. Stated differently, damage to the functionally uncommitted brain is not the same as damage to the committed brain. Based on animal models, there are two major interpretations of the impact of early brain damage. The major premise of the Kennard principle (Kennard, 1940, 1942) is that brain lesions acquired early in life produce fewer deficits than similar lesions sustained in later life. Therefore, the degree of impaired function resulting from brain damage is proportional to the age at which the damage occurred. Conversely, the Dobbing hypothesis (Dobbing & Smart, 1974) holds that brain damage during CNS development has its greatest impact upon those cell populations or processes that show the greatest rate of development at the time of the insult. For example, if an insult occurs during cell division (proliferation), this would result in decreased cell numbers in certain layers within the brain. If the damage was incurred later, when cell differentiation occurred, the result would be alteration of cell size or function (architecture) (e.g., Risser & Edgell, 1988) (see Chapter 4). Because of the sequence of cortical development (including the remodeling, die-back phenomenon), both interpretations are accurate, depending on whether one views the damage on a cellular or a functional level. If damage occurs too early, it will disrupt the actual brain development sequences; later damage will disrupt areas that had been "dedicated" to specific functions. More specifically, the impact of brain damage can be interpreted by integrating both premises: Damage during infancy and early childhood may prove less devastating than damage during the fetal/neonatal period or in the more mature brain (preschool period). Moreover, some researchers suggest that the neural mechanisms underlying novel learning differ from those underlying assimilated skills. If this is the case, the relationship between age/experience and assimilated skills would argue that the balance between these two types of neural mechanisms may be much different in infants and young children than in adults.

Therefore, timing, duration, and type of insult will influence the residual deficits. For example, similar insults may not produce the same neural or neuropsychological dysfunction. A lack of oxygen and a resultant change in blood pH (asphyxia) would produce different neuroanatomical and neurodevelopmental sequelae in full-term and preterm (<37 weeks gestational age) babies. In full-term infants, damage to the outer layers of the cortex could occur (sulci and gyri) increasing the potential for microcephaly. In preterm babies, damage is often deeper within the brain (in the periventricular area) with increased risk for hydrocephalus.

Unfortunately, although determination of etiologies is in the realm of medicine and documentation of consequences is accomplished via neuropsychology, usually it is difficult to determine when the insult occurred. Moreover,

the situation is further complicated by so-called "silent periods"
in which a deficit may show up
early on, disappear, and then reemerge later. Such is the case with
early hypertonia and later learning
problems (Chapter 6). Some damage is not apparent early on, and
the latent effects are not seen until
the functions subserved by the
neural organization and interconnections are tapped (e.g., academics, abstracting skills, sequential
processing). A major premise of
infant and early childhood neuropsychology is that certain types of

Table 1.2. Selective List of Mediating Variables that Influence the Impact of an Etiological Agent on Neural Substrate and Neuropsychological Functioning

Timing, nature, and severity of insult
Age at insult or gestational age at birth
Location, extent, velocity of lesion formation
Plastic, homeostatic, and defense features
Neural commitment
Functional plasticity
Genetic complement
Diagnosis, treatment, and management
Control over secondary consequences of insult
Prevention

Source: Adapted from Risser & Edgell (1988). Used with permission.

neuropsychological dysfunctions are more likely when the child has sustained specific CNS insults. A list of mediating variables that would influence neuropsychological outcome is presented in Table 1.2. Such variables should be considered when the clinician interprets neuropsychological findings.

CONCEPTUAL FRAMEWORKS

It was already noted that a conceptual, neuropsychological framework that could be applied across ages was necessary. To that end, several years ago the author proposed a classification schema for early neuropsychological assessment (Aylward, 1988). This schema was a synthesis of several previous classifications (Levine, 1983; Lezak, 1983), with applicability extended to the neonatal period and early childhood (see Table 1.3). Because neuropsychological assessment must be age specific, all functions are not tested at each age. Some functions (e.g., reflexes, muscle tone) are predominant during the neonatal period, when behavior is less complex and more neurologically oriented. Other functions such as temporal–sequential organization or verbal abstract abilities are not testable until later, coinciding with increased cortical development. Obviously there is much overlap between functions and between classes of functions. This classification schema was applied to 14 different newborn, infant, and toddler/early childhood tests to determine whether or not a particular function was assessed by the specific evaluation instrument (see Aylward, 1988, pp 240–241). The five assessment constructs or item clusters are:

Table 1.3. Classification Schema for Early Neuropsychological Assessment

I. Basic neurological functions/intactness
   Reflexes   Left/right discrepancies
   Asymmetries   Motor inhibition
   Stereotyped/lateralized postures   Protective reflexes
   Muscle tone   Auditory orientation
   Visual tracking/intactness
II. Receptive functions
   Visual perception   Spatial relations
   Auditory/language   Tactile processing
III. Expressive functions
   A. Fine motor/oral motor   B. Gross motor
      Visual-motor integration   Motility
      Language/speech   Coordination
      Fine motor-constructional
      Visual-spatial orientation
      Articulation
IV. Processing
   A. Memory and learning
      Temporal-sequential organization   Anticipatory behaviors
         (auditory)   Visual sequencing
      Visual memory
      Word retrieval
   B. Thinking/reasoning   ·
      Cognitive adaptive (problem solving) Number concepts
      Abstracting (verbal, nonverbal)   Imitation
      Seriation/classification   Judgment
V. Mental activity
   A. Attentional activities/level of consciousness
      Conceptual tracking/concentration Alertness
      Perseveration   Distractibility
      Behavioral states
   B. Activity
      Arousal
      Cognitive
      Motor

Source: Adapted from Aylward (1988). Used with permission.

1   *Basic neurological function/intactness.* This item cluster involves measurement of neurological and functional intactness. Component items such as early reflexes, muscle tone, asymmetries, head control, presence of protective reactions (in response to change in the infant's body orientation in space), and absence of abnormal indicators (e.g., stereotyped movements, excessive drooling, motor overflow) are evaluated. This class of function enables general determination of intactness of the child's CNS.

2   *Receptive functions.* Receptive functions involve the entry of information into the central processing system, utilizing sensation and perception. Visual, auditory, and tactile input are involved, although the first two modalities are emphasized. This class of function becomes more complex with age, and includes verbal receptive items.

3   *Expressive functions.* Expressive functions refer to behaviors produced by the child and observed by the examiner during the evaluation. Three primary functional areas are involved: fine motor (prehension, reaching, eye–hand coordination), oral motor (vocalizations, verbalizations), and gross motor (sitting, crawling, standing, walking, running, jumping). Deficits in this area are often defined as apraxias, dysphasias, anomias, or dyskinesias.

4   *Processing.* Processing includes two components: memory/learning and thinking/reasoning. Therefore, processing involves higher-order functions such as habituation, object permanency, imitation, and problem-solving skills. This area includes coordination of a variety of cognitive processes (e.g., executive and inhibitory), and is considered a good prognostic indicator of an infant's true potential.

5   *Mental activity.* This cluster includes goal directedness, attentional activities, and activity level. These components are more qualitative in nature, and thereby require keen observational skills and familiarity with age-appropriate behavior. This area also involves integration of various brain functions.

These conceptual groupings are not measured equally at each age. In the newborn/neonatal period, neurological function/intactness, gross motor expressive, and mental activity items (state, activity) are predominant; most available tests include these items. In infancy, receptive, expressive, and processing items are emphasized, with particular emphasis being placed on sensorimotor skills. Unfortunately, less attention is given to neurological function/intactness or mental activity items at this age. In the early childhood period, much more emphasis is placed on receptive, expressive, and processing functions, to the general exclusion of neurological function or mental activity clusters (Aylward, 1988, 1994). These conceptual groupings were applied to the Early Neuropsychologic Optimality Rating Scales (ENORS; Aylward, 1988; Aylward, Verhulst & Bell, 1994) (see Chapter 5).

This conceptual framework was altered slightly and provides the basis for the BINS (Aylward, 1995). The five previous clusters were reduced to four, with the Mental Activity and Processing groupings being combined to form Cognitive Processes. The conceptual clusters are not thought to be orthogonal and it is expected that for any given test item, the abilities represented in any one cluster may be primarily involved, although abilities from another cluster could be included as well. For example, when an infant follows commands, both verbal receptive and motor expressive abilities are involved. Similarly, in the case of problem solving with form boards, cognitive processing and receptive functions are important. Therefore, in infant and early childhood neuropsychology, inclusion of an item into one of the conceptual clusters is not a mutually exclusive procedure; many items have a primary conceptual loading on one cluster and a secondary or even tertiary loading on others. Because the complexity of the infant's behavioral repertoire expands significantly over the first several years, there is a lack of absolute continuity in the representativeness of each cluster at each age (see Table 1.4).

These conceptual clusters also provide insight into whether an identified dysfunction is global or more circumscribed and specific. For example, in the case of moderate intraventricular hemorrhage (IVH; see Chapter 4), sequelae are more often manifest in motor rather than higher-order cognitive processes (Lewis & Bendersky, 1989; Selzer, Lindgren, & Blackman, 1992). Therefore, Basic Neurological Function/Intactness items will be affected specifically (such as increased tone in the lower extremities). Item performance on other clusters such as Cognitive Processes might be spared. However, for more severe biological risks such as Stage II or III hypoxic-ischemic encephalopathy (Sarnat & Sarnat, 1976; see Chapter 4), item performance in all four conceptual clusters would likely be negatively affected. A profile of nonoptimal responses that extends across conceptual groupings may indicate gross cognitive deficits, whereas optimal performance on Cognitive Processes items tends to make the prognosis more optimistic (Chapter 6).

■■■■■ SCORING IN INFANT AND EARLY CHILDHOOD NEUROPSYCHOLOGY

The final, introductory issue involves how best to score infant and early childhood neuropsychological test data. Scoring is complex because of the differential

Table 1.4. Primary and Secondary Conceptual Loadings for BINS Items by Age and Item

	Areas of ability			
Age/item	Neurological functions	Receptive functions	Expressive functions	Cognitive processes
3–4 months				
Eyes follow ring		Primary		Secondary
Reaches for suspended ring			Primary	Secondary
5–6 months				
Regards pellet-conjugate gaze	Secondary	Primary		
Uses partial thumb apposition to grasp cube			Primary	Secondary
7–10 months				
Uses pads of fingertips to grasp pellet			Primary	Secondary
Rings bell purposely				Primary
11–15 months				
Removes pellet from bottle				Primary
Puts three cubes in cup			Secondary	Primary
16–20 months				
Imitates crayon stroke			Secondary	Primary
Removes pellet from bottle			Secondary	Primary
21–24 months				
Places three pieces in puzzle board				Primary
Builds tower of six cubes			Primary	Secondary

Source: From Aylward (1995) Bayley Infant Neurodevelopmental Screener Manual, The Psychological Corporation. Reprinted with permission.

emphasis on certain functions at each age. Weighting items and other comparable methods of scoring are not easily adapted to infant and early childhood neuropsychology. Although scoring an individual item or group of related items may not be problematic, it is not clear how individual or even grouped scores could be combined to produce some type of interpretable summary score. This is particularly true when one considers the aforementioned issue of different functions assuming increased or decreased importance, depending on age.

Drawing from the literature on perinatal risk, modifications of two potential scoring procedures were considered in the development of two early developmental neuropsychological tests: ENORS and BINS (Aylward, 1988, 1994, 1995; Aylward, Verhulst, & Bell, 1988a, b, 1992, 1994). In the *complications approach,* points are given cumulatively for the presence of risk factors (i.e., those that would increase the likelihood of compromised development). Complications scales traditionally have been utilized as a means of categorizing children in terms of medical risk. In the alternative *optimality approach*, factors are identified that are most likely to produce positive outcomes; optimality scales have been used for predicting perinatal outcomes (V. J. Molfese, 1989; Prechtl, 1981). Complications scales use weighted values, whereas optimality scales incorporate equal variable weights. However, because nonoptimal conditions rarely occur in isolation, a more serious condition will result in fewer optimal scores with this method (V. J. Molfese, 1989). According to Prechtl's (1981) optimality concept, a normal neurodevelopmental or neuropsychological finding has a higher predictive value for later "normal" functioning than an abnormal sign does for later "abnormal" outcome. The optimality concept should not be considered simply as the reverse of the complications approach. It differs in that the so-called "optimum" sometimes is more narrowly defined than is the range of "normal."

Therefore, several infant neuropsychological assessment instruments (e.g., ENORS, BINS) have incorporated modifications of the premises of the optimality concept. Neuropsychological responses were used instead of the presence or absence of biological risk factors. Rather than focusing on the "normality" or "abnormality" of a particular response, a measure of deviation (or lack of deviation) from an established optimal neuropsychological response, based on a priori decision rules, was determined. Items could simply be scored *optimal* or *nonoptimal* and then summed. The procedure avoids the problem of weighting different items, by allowing these items to be scored as optimal or nonoptimal, and then summed. Cutoff scores (e.g., BINS) or percentage scores (ENORS) could be computed, the latter approach allowing for occasional missing data.

In the case of older children, the conceptual, neuropsychological framework outlined above is still useful (with some modification; see Chapter 5), although the corresponding optimality approach has not received wide application. At this age, the possibility exists that each of the four conceptual groupings or clusters could individually be scored as optimal/nonoptimal based on a priori decisions (versus optimality scorings for individual items within each cluster), so that a profile of the child's areas of strength and difficulty could be determined. Unfortunately, as it now stands, overall scores such as an IQ or DQ (developmental quotient) frequently are misleading, because they do not clarify areas of strengths as well as weaknesses. The global scores become even less meaningful when a later diagnosis such as educable mentally handicapped (EMH) or mild mental retardation is forwarded. Although such a diagnosis might be sufficient for educational purposes in some school systems, early developmental neuropsychology would go a step further and include investigation of the underlying reasons or components for such a score. More specifically, a young child might receive a low score on a standardized, norm-referenced test because of underlying attention, processing, conceptualization, sequencing, or other learning problems. Thus, there is the risk of overgeneralization based on global scores, and inherent in this problem is the strong likelihood of inappropriate or ineffective interventions (e.g., later placement in an EMH class versus one for children with language disorders). Clinicians must look beyond the psychometric data in order to understand the results of infant and early childhood neuropsychological assessment. Systematic observation, task analysis, and error pattern analysis must be employed as well. In addition, assessment instruments often cannot be used interchangeably.

SUMMARY

In summary, infant and early childhood neuropsychology continues to be an evolving discipline. The terms *neuropsychological* and *neurodevelopmental* (and perhaps even *neurobehavioral*) can be used interchangeably at this age (newborn through 5 years) as they consider brain–behavior relationships and combine developmental and neurological approaches. These terms also address biological risk, where the infant's CNS has been exposed to some stressful event. As a result, concurrent and predictive validity are two important concepts in this area. Infant and early childhood neuropsychology differs from other disciplines because of the strong conceptual underpinnings that allow continuity across these early ages, the areas assessed, and interpretation and scoring. Areas of application include, but are not limited to multidisciplinary diagnostic clinics, neonatal intensive care unit follow-up programs, genetics clinics, and other screening and assessment programs for infants and children with drug/alcohol exposure, metabolic disorders, HIV, congenital CNS malformations, acquired brain injury, or other medical conditions.

Because of the interplay between maturation, development, environment, and recovery of function and plasticity, awareness of the contributions of each to "normality" and "abnormality" is critical. The interpretative "mind-set," along with the neuropsychological framework, allows application to existing tests, even though they may not have previously been considered neuropsychological or neurodevelopmental in nature. Finally, this assessment is a "bottom-up" process; one cannot simply scale down tests used for older children or adults. Clinicians must consider that the infant and young child's neuropsychological processes become more qualitatively and quantitatively complex, corresponding to increasing age. Scaling down tests used for older children may address quantitative issues to some degree, but this approach misses the qualitative complexities of the evolving neuroanatomical and behavioral repertoires of the younger child.

The Concept of "Risk" in Infant and Early Childhood Neuropsychology

An important issue in early developmental neuropsychology is the concept of "risk." Tjossem (1976) delineated three categories of risk: *established*, *environmental*, and *biological*. Established risks are medical disorders of a known etiology whose developmental outcome is well documented (e.g., Down syndrome, HIV). Environmental risks include the quality of the mother–infant interaction, opportunities for developmental/cognitive stimulation, and health care. Biological risks include the exposure to potentially noxious prenatal, perinatal, or postnatal developmental events such as asphyxia, intraventricular hemorrhage, and low birth weight (LBW). [LBW is ≤2500 g, very low birth weight (VLBW) is ≤1500 g, and extremely low birth weight (ELBW) is ≤1000 g.] There is increasing interest in infants with birth weights ≤ 800 g (1 lb, 1 oz), who are considered to be at extreme biological risk. Practitioners in infant and early childhood neuropsychology must consider all three categories of risk, with young patients often having more than one type. Although there is continued emphasis on medical factors being causative agents in compromised developmental outcome (Weisglas-Kuperus, Baerts, Smrkovsky, & Sauer, 1993), the importance of environmental risks on later functioning is increasingly recognized (Aylward, 1990, 1992, 1996; Bradley, Whiteside, Mundfrom, & Blevins-Kwabe, 1995).

Established risk is relatively straightforward, and will be discussed further in Chapter 4; the bulk of the present discussion regarding risk will focus on biological and environmental risks. The latter risks often occur together, as children from poor socioeconomic circumstances and poverty are also exposed to medical risk factors such as inadequate prenatal care, LBW, environmental toxins, poor nutrition, drugs, and limited access to medical care. This combination of risks is referred to as *double jeopardy* or *double hazard* (Escalona, 1982; Parker, Greer, & Zuckerman, 1988). In such situations, nonoptimal biological and environmental factors work synergistically to affect outcome negatively. Given that: (1) one in five young children lives in poverty, (2) children at environmental risk are overrepresented in special education classes, and (3) 75% of children with mild mental retardation come from lower-socioeconomic-status (SES) households, clinicians are prone to consider all children from low-SES households to be "at risk" for subnormal intelligence. In actuality, more of these children demonstrate normal, versus deficient, intellectual development. Moreover, four times as many children with IQs less than 70 are born at birth weights ≥ 2500 g, thereby questioning the LBW, biological risk issue. Therefore, in infant and early childhood neuropsychology, the practitioner must be aware of how environmental risks affect neuropsychological findings, and understand the relationships between biological and environmental risks. From at least 12 months onwards, clinicians must consider the results of neuropsychological/neurodevelopmental assessment instruments in conjuction with biological factors *and* environmental influences when determining the need for intervention and in the consideration of possible later outcomes.

ENVIRONMENTAL ISSUES THAT AFFECT NEUROPSYCHOLOGICAL OUTCOMES

Models of Effect

The most accepted model of environmental influence is the *transactional approach* (Sameroff & Chandler, 1975). Here, a degree of plasticity is considered inherent in both the child and the environment. The child is constantly reorganizing and "self-righting": A poorly stimulating environment would interfere with this self-righting, and the probability of a disrupted child–environment transaction increases. A more positive environment is assumed to enhance the child's resiliency. This environmentally driven model has led to coining of the term *continuum of caretaking casualty*. A variation of this model is the *risk route* concept (Aylward & Kenny, 1979), which requires assessment of the child at various times in three areas: medical/biological, environmental/psychosocial, and behavioral/developmental. The degree of risk is additive across the three areas at each time of assessment, and is cumulative over time. It is highly recommended that these three interrelated areas always be considered in early neuropsychological assessment.

Specific Environmental Factors

SES is represented by maternal education and occupational status. Social support includes tangible (housing, financial assistance) and intangible (attitudes, encouragement, family practices regarding academics) components. The environment also includes "process" and "status" features. The former are specific aspects of the environment that are experienced directly (objects, persons, events), whereas status factors are broader and are experienced more indirectly (social class, location of residence). Process factors are considered more *proximal* in that they involve the child and caretakers on a regular basis (e.g., mother–infant interaction). Status factors are *distal*, meaning they are secondary and more peripheral. The effects of status variables such as SES and maternal education become increasingly apparent between 18 and 36 months of age, with 24 months being an age cited frequently (Aylward, 1990, 1992). However, environmental effects are apparent even during the first year of life. Process variables (e.g., parent–child interaction) are better *early* predictors of certain types of neuropsychological and cognitive outcomes; generalized, distal measures are more predictive if measured later. Moreover, single or isolated negative environmental factors have a small, incremental effect on later cognitive functioning; it is the *accumulation* of risk factors that is the major contributor to neurodevelopmental morbidity (Sameroff, Seifer, Barocas, Zax, & Greenspan, 1987). The presence of poverty increases the likelihood that personal or situational determinants of parenting will become risk factors rather than protective factors in the child's life. Thus, the chronic and pervasive influence of poverty increases the probability that the negative impact of early environmental (and biological) risk factors will accumulate and persist over time, increasing the strong draw toward a poor neuropsychological outcome.

Specific Neuropsychological Processes

Environmental variables most strongly influence verbal and general cognitive outcome, whereas medical/biological factors are more strongly related to neurological and perceptual-performance functions (Aylward et al., 1994). Medical/biological factors may influence cognitive scores if the tests include perceptual-performance and, perhaps, memory items. These findings suggest that the verbal expressive and receptive neuropsychological item clusters noted previously, as well as cognitive processes, would potentially be influenced by environmental variables. Basic neurological functions, gross and fine motor expressive, and visual and auditory (but not verbal) receptive items would be relatively unaffected by negative environmental influences. Conversely, motor and sensory receptive neuropsychological functions would be affected by biological risks.

Relationship between Biological and Environmental Risks

It is apparent that biological and environmental risks work in tandem to affect neuropsychological outcome. These factors are highly interrelated, and the relationship becomes complex, considering the aforementioned fact that low-SES children also have more biological risks such as perinatal complications and LBW. Biological risk factors tend to be associated with severe mental retardation and multiple handicaps, and when biological risk is severe, the mediating influence of the environment is reduced. Environmental (and possibly genetic) factors are assumed to be the underlying cause of mild mental retardation (sometimes called *familial* or *sociocultural mental retardation*), because biological factors other than genetics cannot be identified, and most mildly mentally retarded children live in lower-SES households (Shonkoff, 1982). Biological factors also determine whether a given neurodevelopmental dysfunction or deficit will occur. Environmental factors have a tempering effect and determine the severity (again, except in cases of severe biological risk) (Hunt, Cooper, & Tooley, 1988). Vis-à-vis the transactional or risk route approaches, a positive environment seems to facilitate the self-righting tendencies of the child, thereby enhancing neuropsychological resiliency to biological stresses.

Recently, it has been questioned whether it is the environment that exerts a cumulative, negative effect on later outcome, or whether declines in later functioning are the manifestations of an insidious genetic influence. Data from the Texas Adoption Project (Loehlin, 1989) indicate that environmental effects are influential early in childhood, but have a decreasing influence on IQ as children grow older. Changes in genetic expression continue into late adolescence or early adulthood. It is also possible that prenatal stressors faced by the mother may affect fetal brain development, such as the "fetal stress syndrome" (Lou, Hanson, Nordentoft, & Pryds, 1994), in which small head circumferences have been reported. These children also have demonstrated suboptimal neonatal neurological scores (Prechtl, 1977). These prenatal biological influences (e.g., glucocorticoids) could be misinterpreted as genetic influences.

Recently, data on 350 pairs of twins from the MacArthur Longitudinal Twin Study (Cherny et al., 1994) indicated the presence of substantial genetic continuity (40% heritability) of general cognitive ability from 14 to 24 months. However, significant, new genetic variation also appeared at 24 months. Shared environmental influences increased sharply from 14 to 24 months, from about 20% to 40%. Therefore, although the shared environmental influences and genetics contribute to continuity of mental development, it is possible that new, genetically influenced developmental processes occur at the transition from infancy to early childhood. These data are intriguing, and also underscore the important role of behavioral genetics in early developmental neuropsychology.

Therefore, at early ages, "process" or proximal factors (e.g., early mother–child interactions) will be influential regarding neurodevelopmental functioning (in addition to genetic influences). During the toddler and early school age periods, "status" or distal factors (e.g., SES) will become more important. In late childhood and early adolescence, genetic factors again will provide additional influence.

IMPLICATIONS

Practitioners in the field of infant and early childhood neuropsychology must consider how "risks," whether established, biological, environmental, or in some combination, influence assessment data. Certain types of risks will have specific influences. There appears to be direct linkage between both (1) established risks (genetic syndromes) and (2) severe biological risks, and later, severe neurodevelopmental dysfunctions such as cerebral palsy, epilepsy, mental retardation (moderate to severe), and neurosensory disorders (e.g., blindness, hearing impairment). There are accumulating data indicating that less debilitating, *high-prevalence/low-severity dysfunctions* (Levine, 1983) also are associated with biological risks. These high-prevalence/low-severity dysfunctions include learning disabilities, behavior disorders, and attention deficit disorders. Biological risks determine whether a deficit will occur, but environmental factors will modulate severity, unless the degree of biological risk and the resulting CNS disruption is severe. In such cases, biological influences place a "ceiling" on neuropsychological/cognitive functioning that essentially precludes any mediating environmental effects. Vis-à-vis the transactional and risk route models, an infant's intrinsic developmental vulnerability can be moderated by the influence of extrinsic (environmental) protective factors that increase the probability of positive adaptation.

Motor, neurological, and perceptual-performance functions are most susceptible to biological risks. Verbal and cognitive functions are more strongly influenced by environmental risks. The influence of environmental risks increases between 18 and 24 months of age. Therefore, correlations between cognitive scores and environment increase with age, whereas correlations between cognitive scores and biological variables correspondingly decrease as the child gets older. Because of these relationships, motor and neurological functions have been found to be relatively stable over a 3-year span in biologically at-risk infants (Aylward, Gustafson, Verhulst, & Colliver, 1987), while cognitive function (which is affected by environmental risks) can decline dramatically. More specifically, in a recent study, 9 out of 10 children with normal motor or neurological function at 9 months continued to have normal function at 36 months. However, 25% of children who had normal cognitive function at 9 months did not have normal McCarthy Scales of Children's Abilities (McCarthy, 1972) General Cognitive Indexes (GCIs) at 36 months (Aylward et al., 1987). Of note is the fact that GCI contains neuropsychological perceptual-performance and quantitative items. In a different sample, memory functions also were associated with biological risks (Aylward, 1993). Therefore, the type of assessment measure is critical, and one must consider that most neuropsychological tests involve verbal and cognitive items as well as those that tap perceptual-performance, quantitative, memory, and attention constructs.

The combination of biological and environmental risks appears particularly devastating for a child's outcome. Hunt et al. (1988) followed a sample of 108 LBW infants for 8 years and found that of children from families with low parental education (environmental risk) and high neonatal illness (biological risk), more than 55% had moderate to severe developmental dysfunction. In contrast, only 9% of children with high neonatal illness but from families with high parental education had similar problems. This again underscores the negative influences of double jeopardy.

It also is quite possible that environment and established risk have a similar, interactive relationship. *Behavioral phenotypes* are behavior patterns associated with identifiable syndromes and are not learned characteristics of the disorder (e.g., eating problems in Prader–Willi syndrome). Although these behaviors have a genetic basis, they can be modified by the environment (but remain characteristic of the syndrome). In other words, the "penetrance" is affected by environmental factors. The term, *ecogenetic* may be applicable in this situation (J. C. Harris, 1995). Clinicians also should consider the fact that identical behavioral phenotypes may have heterogeneous bases (as in the case of autism).

Biological and environmental risks will affect the findings of neuropsychological evaluations, and these findings will drive the focus of interventions. Parry (1992) delineated three groups of infants and young children who receive interventions: (1) those at environmental risk (the largest group), (2) those at increased biological risk, and (3) infants with established developmental delays, disabilities, or deviations. Thus, the type of risk will affect the type of assessment findings, which in turn will determine the type of intervention. Interventions are most effective if they are multifaceted, delivered early, and the child has mild to moderate problems. Interventions may not necessarily enhance a given child's outcome to an average or above-average level, but rather may prevent further, slow decline away from average. Emphasis should be placed on enhancement of verbal and cognitive functioning in particular, as these areas are most susceptible to negative environmental influences (Aylward, 1996). In regard to neuropsychological functioning, there is broad theoretical support for the notion that intrinsic developmental vulnerability can be moderated by the influence of extrinsic (environmental) protective factors that increase the probability of positive adaptation. Genetic influences may also drive development by influencing the child's early responses to the environment in terms of the child eliciting interaction and seeking experiences.

In terms of application, infant and early childhood neuropsychologists must consider the results of neuropsychological tests in conjunction with the degree of biological and environmental risk. For example, assume that the clinician administers the BINS (Aylward, 1995) to a 2-year-old from an upper-SES, highly stimulating environment, and finds nonoptimal performance on language (expressive and receptive) and cognitive processes items. Concern then is raised that there is underlying cognitive dysfunction and limitation. In this case, environmental risk is minimal and therefore could not explain the poor performance in areas traditionally strongly associated with environmental influences. Biological and/or established risk influences should be considered. Additional assessment instruments should be administered. However, directing intervention to enhance environmental quality is questionable. Conversely, if this child came from a poor, uneducated, single-parent household that provided minimal stimulation, then consideration of influential factors might change, and intervention might be geared more toward improvement of environmental circumstances.

In a different case, assume that the clinician administers the BINS to a 6-month-old (age corrected for prematurity) girl, born at 25 weeks gestational age and who experienced a variety of perinatal difficulties, including respiratory distress syndrome, Grade II intraventricular hemorrhage (see Chapter 4), and other typical problems of prematurity (e.g., apnea, hyperbilirubinemia, retinopathy of prematurity). Evaluation revealed problems in neurological functions/intactness and expressive motor functions items, with increased axial tone (torso) and increased tone of the lower extremities (legs). Optimal performance was obtained on cognitive processes (precursory object permanency, goal-directed behaviors) and fine motor and language expressive functions (vocalizes). In this case, the type of neuropsychological dysfunction more likely can be attributed to biological risk. Moreover, knowledge of the relationships between neuropsychological findings and specific risk status would assist the clinician in explaining findings to parents, determining the best type of intervention (e.g., occupational and physical therapy), and in terms of prognostic implications.

Development of the Central Nervous System

In the practice of infant and early childhood neuropsychology, it is not unusual for the clinician to encounter problems such as microcephaly, hydrocephalus, myelomeningocele, and other brain abnormalities. Similarly, abnormalities of the skin and hair or dysmorphic facial features can heighten the concern for underlying CNS anomalies. In essence, to appreciate abnormalities in brain function and their clinical significance, infant and early childhood neuropsychologists should be well versed in their understanding of *normal* CNS development and related concepts. Information about CNS development is useful in identifying potential causes of cognitive or neurodevelopmental dysfunction, and knowledge of the relationships between certain brain anomalies and neuropsychological findings helps to guide clinicians' diagnostic sensitivity. This chapter contains a brief summary of pre-, peri- and postnatal CNS development. The discussion focuses on the CNS (brain and spinal cord), as distinct from the peripheral nervous system (nerves leading from the spinal cord to peripheral structures) or the autonomic nervous system (nerves controlling visceral functions).

CRITICAL AND SENSITIVE PERIODS

Clarification of the concepts of *critical period* and *sensitive period* is necessary. The former is the time during which the action of a specific internal or external influence is necessary (critical) for normal developmental progress (Capone, 1996). In contrast, the latter is the time during which the CNS is highly susceptible to the effects of harmful or deleterious internal or external conditions. Therefore, a critical period occurs when certain conditions are necessary for the CNS to develop *normally*; a sensitive period is the time in which damage to the CNS can lead to *alterations, reorganization, and potential aberrations* of the system. Critical periods can be viewed as being more discrete, whereas sensitive periods are on more of a continuum and therefore are less rigid.

CNS MATURATION ━━━

For purposes of simplicity, maturation of the CNS may be divided into six major developmental events: (1) dorsal induction, (2) ventral induction, (3) neuronal proliferation, (4) neuronal migration, (5) organization/differentiation (axonal and dendritic growth, synaptogenesis, cell/axonal death), and (6) myelination (Capone, 1996; Hallett & Proctor, 1996; J. C. Harris, 1995; Lyon & Gadisseux, 1991; Volpe, 1987). Lyon and Gadisseux (1991) suggested that prenatal brain development may be broadly conceptualized as consisting of two major phases. In the first phase, spanning the initial 20 weeks of fetal life, organogenesis, neuronogenesis, and neuronal migration occur; the second phase (from 20 to 40 weeks) is characterized by neuronal growth and maturation.

The developmental organization of the CNS is the result of a multitude of well-choreographed processes that involve complex biochemical and cellular mechanisms. These occur in a precisely ordered and timed sequence. Each process is partially dependent on the result or outcome of related, preceding events, and the entire developmental scheme is genetically determined (e.g., Capone, 1996; J. C. Harris, 1995).

PRINCIPLES OF NEURAL DEVELOPMENT ━━━━━━━━━━━━━━━━━━━━━━━━━━━━━

Capone (1996) and others have delineated principles of neural development that are of interest to clinicians and researchers in early developmental neuropsychology. Selected general principles are:

1	Neurodevelopment depends on genetic and epigenetic (one stage builds upon another) influences.
2	Formation of brain regions is precisely timed, with more primitive and caudal parts (e.g., brainstem) being formed before more complex and highly evolved structures (cerebral cortex).
3	Within the cortex, neurons that appear earlier in development occupy deeper layers than those generated later.
4	The immature brain receives environmental input and responds in terms of differentiation (see Chapter 2).
5	Brain growth varies by region, and these regions are most vulnerable when they are most rapidly growing.
6	The lineage of specific cell types in many primitive animals is largely preordained; in complex animals (e.g., humans), the fate of individual cells is more flexible (allowing for plasticity).
7	Cell position is an important component of the epigenetic influences on differentiation.

8	As neurons mature, they acquire obligatory trophic (growth) dependencies on other cells for input, nourishment, and other needs.
9	Nerve terminals compete with each other for trophic support.
10	The sphere of influences that act on the CNS continually expands during development.
11	Because of its prolonged period of development, the brain is the most vulnerable of all embryonic/fetal organs to teratologic insult.
12	Birth does not mark a particular milestone in the biological development of the brain.
13	There is no simple, one-to-one relationship between a cause and the final morphological appearance of the brain.
14	The developmental timing of an insult may be more important than the nature of the insult itself in determining the pattern of malformation.
15	Functions that are localized to discrete regions of the brain are the elementary operations, rather than the complex faculties.
16	Complex faculties are constructed from serial and parallel connections among several brain regions; interrelated brain functions are not a series of links in a single chain.

MAJOR DEVELOPMENTAL EVENTS IN CNS MATURATION

Dorsal Induction (3–4 weeks gestation)

This is the first stage of CNS development. In the developing embryo, the neural plate evolves from a thickened area of the ectoderm and produces neurons and glial cells. The neural ectoderm then folds back to form a neural tube, the precursor of the brain and spinal cord (Fig. 3.1). The cavity of the neural tube produces the ventricular system, and the neuroepithelium produces the neurons and glial cells. The caudal (posterior or back) part of the neural tube produces the spinal cord; the rostral (anterior or front) section evolves into the brain. Further elongation, folding, and thickening of the neural tube (changes in the longitudinal and circumferential dimensions of the straight, "pipelike" structure) produce the six divisions of the CNS. By day 25, three primary brain vesicles are apparent: (1) the prosencephalon (forebrain vesicle), (2) the mesencephalon (midbrain vesicle), and (3) the rhombencephalon (hindbrain vesicle).

By day 32, the prosencephalon and the rhombencephalon divide in two. The former divides into the telencephalon and the diencephalon, and the latter divides into the metencephalon and the myelencephalon. A detailed chronology of human brain development is given by Rubenstein, Lotspeich, and Ciaranello (1990). The

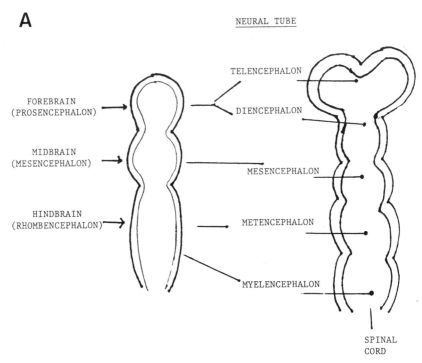

A

NEURAL TUBE

FOREBRAIN
(PROSENCEPHALON)

TELENCEPHALON

DIENCEPHALON

MIDBRAIN
(MESENCEPHALON)

MESENCEPHALON

HINDBRAIN
(RHOMBENCEPHALON)

METENCEPHALON

MYELENCEPHALON

SPINAL
CORD

Figure 3.1. Nervous system development. (A) Schematic of three- and five-vesicle stages. (B) Flexures (bends) and resultant vesicles.

sequence of development from the three-vesicle stage, to the five-vesicle stage, to the mature CNS derivatives is outlined in Table 3.1. Abnormalities at this time result in disorders of neural tube closure such as myelomeningocele, anencephaly, encephalocele, or profoundly impaired neuropsychological function (see Chapter

Table 3.1. Sequence of CNS Development

Three-vesicle stage	Five-vesicle stage	Mature structure
Forebrain (prosencephalon)	Telencephalon	Cerebral cortex, basal ganglia, hippocampus, amygdala, olfactory bulbs
	Diencephalon	Thalamus, hypothalamus, optical tracts, retinae
Midbrain (mesencephalon)	Mesencephalon	Midbrain
Hindbrain (rhombencephalon)	Metencephalon	Pons, cerebellum
	Myelencephalon	Medulla oblongata
Caudal part of neural tube	Same	Spinal cord

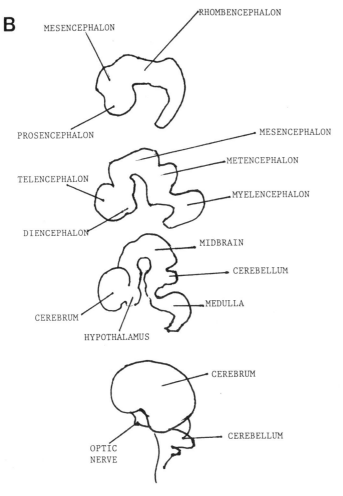

B

MESENCEPHALON

RHOMBENCEPHALON

PROSENCEPHALON

MESENCEPHALON

TELENCEPHALON

METENCEPHALON

MYELENCEPHALON

DIENCEPHALON

MIDBRAIN

CEREBELLUM

MEDULLA

CEREBRUM

HYPOTHALAMUS

CEREBRUM

CEREBELLUM

OPTIC
NERVE

Figure 3.1. (*Continued*).

4). Because the neural plate and skin both evolve from the ectoderm layer of embryonic tissue, there is a link between skin lesions and brain conditions such as tuberous sclerosis or neurofibromatosis ("neurocutaneous" syndromes).

Ventral Induction (5–6 weeks gestation)

The ventral induction process marks the second stage of CNS development during which the major portion of the brain (the cerebrum) and the face are formed. A series of cleavages divide the cerebrum into the left and right hemispheres. Cleavage along the horizontal plane results in paired optic vesicles, olfactory bulbs, and tracts. Essentially, this process reflects segmentation of the neural tube along its longitudinal axis. It is assumed that the homeobox genes, a specific subclass of developmentally regulated genes, are important in determining boundaries between adjacent vesicles (Capone, 1996). Ventral induction also produces the cerebellum. Therefore, the basic structural subdivisions are formed by the end of the first 6 weeks of gestation. Interference at this time results in failure of the brain to make the appropriate cleavages, causing holoprosencephaly, seizures, and/or profound neurological/neuropsychological impairment. In addition, involvement of the midline facial structures including the eyes, nose, and mouth often occurs, resulting in dysmorphic facial appearance. This helps to explain why certain facial abnormalities can be indicative of structural CNS abnormalities.

Proliferation (2–4 months peak time of occurrence)

Although proliferation begins as early as the first or second month of gestation, as the fetal period begins more dramatic growth occurs in the radial dimension of the brain vesicles, particularly the wall of the telencephalic vesicle from which the cerebral cortex arises. The cortex first expands rostrally to form the frontal lobes, then dorsally to form the parietal lobes. The cortex then expands posteriorly and inferiorly to form the temporal and occipital lobes. Neuroblasts (precursors of nerve cells) proliferate (via mitosis) to create the lifetime number (100 billion) of neurons (nerve cells) that the individual will possess. Proliferation increases exponentially through the first half of gestation (20 weeks) and continues into the second and third postnatal years before leveling off. The first distinct phase is between 10 and 20 weeks, with the principal neurons being generated in the germinal matrix within the ventricular zone. Smaller interneurons appear to have a less well-defined and more protracted time course of proliferation. The principal neurons are those with large axons that form major pathways (Golgi class I); the interneurons (sometimes called *microneurons*) form connections within brain areas (Golgi class II). Neurons found in the deeper layers of the cortex are created before those in outer layers. Therefore, most neurons are generated by the final trimester; subsequently, there is primarily glial cell proliferation. The number of neurons created during proliferation is 40–50% more than is needed in the mature brain. This redundancy will resolve during differentiation. The second major proliferative phase begins at 4–5 months postnatally and is associated with glial cell multiplication (Capone, 1996; J. C. Harris, 1995). In general, growth varies in different regions of the brain, and these various regions are most vulnerable to disruption when they are most rapidly growing. Although no new neurons are created once the stage of proliferation culminates (they are irreplaceable), functional reorganization of existing neuron populations to supplement or even assume the responsibilities of other neurons can occur. The inability to generate new neurons once proliferation is complete might at first appear to be a disadvantage; however, it has been argued that the addition of new, "naive" neurons into existing, functional cortical circuits would interfere with retention of learned behaviors and acquired experiences. Therefore, the cessation of neuronal generation may, in actuality, be an advantage. Abnormalities at this time can result in microcephaly (head size greater than 2 SDs below average), or megalencephaly (macrocephaly), and can also lead to mental retardation and other anomalies.

Migration (3–5 months)

Migration refers to the movement of nerve cells from their sites of origin (ventricular zone) to their final positions. These events transform the four fundamental embryonic layers of the telencephalic wall into the six-layered structure of the adult cerebral cortex. There are two waves of neuronal migration to the cortical plate, occurring at 8–10 and 11–15 weeks gestation, respectively. Young neurons migrate in sheets (laminae) of similar cells toward specific zones in the outer layer of the neural tube, which will become the multilayered cortical *gray matter* and subcortical nuclei. Axons that connect this layer to target synapses form an intermediate layer known as *white matter*.

The earliest-generated neurons occupy the deep cortical layers, whereas those generated later in gestation will reside in more superficial layers. Thus, the cerebral cortex basically is developed in an "inside-out" manner, from layer VI (deepest) to layer I. Newly formed neurons glide along radial glial fibers that serve as a passive "guide wire" to the periphery, from the germinal layer out to the cortex. Neurons destined for later layers must migrate through earlier, deeper layers. Migration is vulnerable to genetic disturbances, viral infections, and vascular disruptions. In some fashion (probably genetic), each neuron acquires positional information that establishes its local address with the cortical plate. The different layers contain different types of neurons and neurotransmitters. In addition to being organized horizontally in layers, the cerebral cortex is also organized vertically in "ontogenetic" columns, thereby making columns functional units. Cells within a cortical column share functional features that are distinct from cells in adjacent columns. Columns are linked together by specific sets of input–output connections, and each column spans the width of the cerebral cortex. During the fifth month of gestation, the cerebral convolutions first appear, namely, sulci (groovelike depressions) and gyri (elevations or ridges). Secondary and tertiary sulci appear between 7 and 9 months gestation; most gyri are present by 28 weeks.

Neural abnormalities that may occur during this phase include bilateral cleft of the cerebral hemispheres with incomplete formation of all six layers (schizencephaly), smooth brain surface with too few or too many gyri, or abnormal gyri and sulci (lissencephaly, agyria, pachygyria, or microgyria), agenesis of the corpus callosum, and neurons in abnormal locations (neuronal hereotopias). See Chapter 4. The type of disorder depends on the timing of the neuronal migration disruption.

Organization/Differentiation (6 months gestation–5 years)

Once neurons reach their destination, they begin to grow and differentiate (cytodifferentiation). Usually, sheets of neurons express their distinctive morphological and biochemical phenotypes (differentiation), and arrange themselves into an extensive network of functioning circuits (organization).

Axonal and Dendritic Growth

Initially, young neurons emit fibrous processes, called *neurites*, that will become axons and dendrites. Axons are *presynaptic* (send messages), whereas dendrites are *postsynaptic* (receive messages), thereby determining polarity and later connectivity. Axonal and dendritic outgrowth is called *morphological differentiation*. During neuronal differentiation, the axon is the first outgrowth to distinguish itself. *Connectivity* consists of axonal pathfinding and target recognition, with subsequent dendritic arborization (branching) and spine formation (neuropil). The number of spines increases with age during development. The synapse comprises presynaptic and postsynaptic elements that allow neurons to communicate with one another using chemical signals. A *cleft* separates the axon and dendrite so that they are not in direct contact. Synapses first make their appearance within the cortical plate by 23 weeks gestation. Synapses are overproduced early in development (up to 2–3 years of age) and then are selectively eliminated or "screened" at a later time (e.g., by adolescence synaptic density is about 60% of the maximum seen at 2 years of age). The strategy of redundancy during the formation of neural connections is probably designed to ensure innervation of all available targets as promptly as possible. "Hardwiring" of neural structures is the rule in phylogenetically older regions of the brain involved in basic regulatory processes (e.g., brain stem), probably allowing for immediate adaptation to the environment (yet simultaneously restricting behavioral plasticity). "Softwiring" is found in phylogenetically more recent areas of the brain (neocortex) and allows for learning and plasticity.

Cell Death

Synaptic survival may in part be dependent on functional stimulation of neurons via sensory and motor input, according to a "use it or lose it" condition. In addition to the large number of synaptic connections that disappear (*pruning*), many cells also are eliminated. Besides the loss due to lack of use, cell death may also be genetically programmed. Retrograde axonal transport of nerve growth factor (NGF) from a target cell back to a cell body may also play a role in survival or death of cells that may or may not have been successful in reaching their target. It is also possible that genetic disorders may cause an imbalance between programs sustaining cells and those causing cell death. Programmed cell death (*apoptosis*) is critical, as death of excessive neurons is necessary for sculpting and fine-tuning the brain. The neural network structures that have survived pruning and cell die-back maintain some plasticity in response to experience.

BRAIN METABOLISM

Brain imaging studies such as positron emission tomography (PET) and single-photon emission tomography (SPECT) enable measurement of local cerebral metabolic rates for glucose. These glucose metabolism rates differ in neonates and adults. In the newborn, the areas of highest activity include the primary sensorimotor cortex, thalamic nuclei, brain stem, and cerebellar vermis (Chugani, 1993). Metabolic activity in the frontal lobes is low between 2 and 4 months and this is the last region to show maturational increases in local glucose metabolism (at 8–12 months). Increases in glucose metabolism at 2–3 months correspond to suppression of subcortical reflexes and maturation of visuo-sensorimotor integration. Increases in local glucose metabolism at 8–9 months in the frontal and associative regions correspond to cognitive development milestones such as object permanency, imitation, and problem solving. Glucose metabolism increases to the adult level by the second year, and exceeds adult rates from ages 3–9 years. This increase is thought to reflect excessive activity resulting from the rapid overproduction of synapses. Subsequently, brain activity and concomitant glucose metabolism decrease until adolescence, when they once again reach adult levels. These findings further support the position that pruning and die-back result in fewer but more efficient neural circuits. Of interest also is the fact that brain plasticity appears to decrease, corresponding to decreases in glucose metabolism.

In terms of neurodevelopmental disorders, impaired dendritic arborization and dendritic spine dysgenesis are associated with mental retardation and seizures. Neuropsychologists should also consider that biochemical differentiation of young neurons occurs in conjunction with morphological differentiation.

Neurotransmitter synthesis, storage, degradation, and receptors all have a developmental sequence. These changes will not be described here, and the reader is referred to Capone (1996) for further reading.

Myelination (6 months gestation to adulthood)

Myelination begins at 6 months gestation. Glial cells produce myelin, a fatty sheath, that eventually covers and insulates many axons, providing for rapid, more efficient impulse transmission. Prior to myelination, neuronal communication is slow, with long refractory periods (speeds increase from 1–2 mps to 50–100 mps). Not all neuronal populations require myelination. In fact, new glia and myelin are the prime factors that account for postnatal growth. At birth the brain weighs approximately 350 g, and at age 2, 1300 g (adult weight is 1400–1500 g). As already mentioned, the area of the brain that contains many bundles of myelinated axons is referred to as *white matter.*

MYELINATION "RULES"

There are several general rules regarding myelination: (1) Proximal pathways myelinate before distal pathways, (2) sensory pathways myelinate before motor pathways, and (3) projection pathways myelinate before association pathways. Myelination progresses from the central sulcus outward toward the occipital, frontal, and temporal poles. For example, pyramidal tract efferents (transmitting outwards) from the motor cortex are myelinated by the end of the first year. However, association cortex interneurons (Golgi class II) complete myelination from late infancy through middle childhood (see Yakovlev & Le Cours, 1967, for further review). Similarly, the midbrain corticovisual pathways necessary for the visual-smile response are myelinated at 2–3 months, and fine motor coordination development corresponds to myelination. Myelination of the frontal lobes proceeds into early adulthood. An interesting table relating changes in myelination and glucose metabolism to language development and Piagetian stages can be found in Hallett and Proctor (1996). Deficient myelin production or presence is associated with cerebral white matter hypoplasia, amino acid defects, organic acid defects, or degenerative diseases (Chapter 4).

NEUROPSYCHOLOGICAL IMPLICATIONS

As has been suggested, infant and early childhood neuropsychology contains the assumption that psychological processes are based in, and arise out of, neurological functions in the CNS (Anastasiow, 1990). Therefore, there is significant overlap with psychobiology. In infant and early childhood neuropsychology, however, the influence of extrinsic factors (environmental experiences) on CNS development is more important than at other ages.

FUNCTIONAL ORGANIZATION

Differentiation and myelination are paralleled by elaboration of the infant's and child's adaptive behavioral repertoire (as in the case of the visual-smile response or fine motor coordination). Structural changes produce modifications in behavior, yet simultaneously, brain structures are influenced by behavioral experiences and the environment. In fact, Risser and Edgell (1988) suggested that assessment of young children depends on measures that take into account the pattern of structural and functional maturation. As a result, the behavioral geography of the brain in infants and young children cannot be viewed in the same manner as that of the adult.

A critical question regarding the interface between environmental learning and CNS development concerns the best time for environmental learning to occur (Anastasiow, 1990). More specifically, should environmental input and stimulation occur before the brain matures sufficiently to mediate the skill in question, or should input occur after sufficient brain maturation? It appears that there are critical times before maturation (myelination) in which experiences should happen, when the brain is most open to such input (i.e., plastic). Experiences that enhance and are necessary for sensory development should occur during early periods in brain growth if the sensory systems are to function optimally. It is in these early periods that the brain is most receptive to extrinsic environmental experiences. Moreover, the sensory systems become established and fully mature during this early brain period.

TYPES OF SYNAPSES

Greenough and Juraska (1986) identified two types of synapses that become evident during the period of rapid synapse proliferation: *experience-expectant* and *experience-dependent* synapses. Expectant synapses are genetically programmed to be ready to receive experiences (input) that are adaptive, species specific, and highly likely to occur. Environmental experiences cause the neurons to be activated and continued neuronal activation stabilizes and makes persistent connections or circuits. Death (pruning) occurs for unused synapses. Synapse stabilization enables the infant to store experience from the environment, and these synapses develop into neural structures that are components of functioning brain systems. Dependent synapses are not genetically programmed, but develop independently from unique environmental experiences; they are generated as the child receives novel experiences. These synapses are produced throughout the individual's lifetime, provided the structures in which they develop retain some degree of plasticity. These can also be generated as a result of insult to the brain. Therefore, early input will "prime" the expectant synapses, and also facilitate development of input-dependent synapses.

Hubel and Wiesel's (1970) landmark animal studies further underscore these principles. During the first 8 weeks of life, the kitten's visual system is very plastic and ready to respond to and develop visual structures from extrinsic patterned light. Kittens deprived of light during these first 8 weeks act as if they are functionally blind, despite relatively normal visual systems. Thus, the presence of the extrinsic light is critical for the development of sight, and without this experience, the neurons in the visual area apparently fail to transmit to other brain areas. Moreover, these animals tend to develop structures that are viewed as abnormal, which will cause irreversible changes if not corrected. Irreversibility occurs because of the effect of the abnormal visual input on the pattern of synapse organization. In this case, experience is recorded in species-specific, "unexpected" ways, and following the period of plasticity, synapses that could have been used to establish normal vision will have been lost. This phenomenon has been replicated in human infants with strabismus (where one eye cannot focus in conjunction with the other as a result of problems with the eye musculature). Here, surgical correction should occur before 4 years of age, as this is the critical period for development of the visual system. In fact, recently some ophthalmologists have performed this surgery in the first several months of life, because of the negative effect uncorrected strabismus has on the subsequent organization of the visual system.

Relating back to critical periods, these appear to be determined by genetically programmed release of *neurotransmitters* (Greenough & Juraska, 1986) and it is at these times that the brain is most receptive to particular experiences. The critical period is indicated by "fixed-action patterns" or "fixed-behavior patterns." The social smile is a reflexive, fixed-behavior pattern that occurs at approximately 2–3 months. If it is cued by a return smile from a caretaker, then it will become stabilized and remain. However, in an infant with visual impairment, the smile may not persist unless cued by auditory or haptic stimulation. Similarly, cooing and babbling will occur even in deaf infants, but if there is no visual or haptic input in response to the infant's vocalization, this fixed-behavior pattern will extinguish. Therefore, the emergence of initial fixed-behavior patterns is genetically prewired or programmed. Whether these behaviors will persist depends on extrinsic input.

Clinicians should also be aware that different brain systems mature at different rates. For example, there are major periods of growth in visual tract myelination between 2–3 and 7–9 months (Lecours, 1975). However, the auditory system does not achieve a level of maturation comparable to the 2- to 3-month visual system until 7–9 months. The auditory system at 4–5 years of age is as mature as the visual system was at 7–9 months (Lecours, 1975). Therefore, the auditory system has a longer period of plasticity than does the visual system. This myelogenetic cycle can explain neuropsychological landmarks as well (Fischer & Pipp, 1984). Pathways in the brain stem and limbic system develop during the first 6 months, pathways in the cortex myelinate from birth to 5 years, and association pathways develop from the first several months through late adolescence. These developments coincide with neurodevelopmental milestones such as crying and cooing, babbling, expressive jargon and word imitation, production of first words, and then word combinations.

The relationship between function and maturation is also evident in the work of Luria (1973). In this framework, cortical function is divided into three zones: *primary, secondary,* and *tertiary.* Primary zones are modality specific and receive direct input from the senses or control motor activity (afferent layer IV). These are fully functional by the end of the first year. Secondary zones integrate modality-specific information into perceptive information (layers II and III), and are fully functional by age 5 years. Tertiary zones are the associative, supramodal areas involving the parietal, temporal, occipital, and prefrontal areas. These zones integrate across modalities and perform executive, purposive, and higher-order cognitive functions. Tertiary zones are functional by 5–8 years of age. Interestingly, maturation of these zones corresponds to Piaget's stages of cognitive development.

There is a hierarchical relationship of zones and lateralization of function. Therefore, the ability to assess various neuropsychological functions is dependent to a significant degree on the stage of functional development of the particular underlying cortical structure. This is a critical distinction that once again separates infant and early childhood neuropsychology from adult neuropsychology. Moreover, functions are processed through many neuronal pathways that are parallel in distribution; complex faculties are constructed from serial and parallel connections among several brain regions. Therefore, early damage to a single area does not necessarily result in the disappearance or maldevelopment of a specific later mental function. Partial return may occur by continued development or reorganization of undamaged parts of the brain. It is not the individual function, but the integration of functional units that is critical to efficient neuropsychological operations. For this reason, early measures that tap discrete functions may not be good predictors of later neuropsychological outcome. Instead, measures such as the Cognitive Processes or Receptive and Expressive

Language items on the BINS (or similar instruments) that involve coordination of several functional units, provide the best "window" to later functioning. Neural tissue can respond to damage not only by creating new synapses to aid in recovery of function, but also by changing the nature of their preprogrammed function.

4

Disorders in Brain Development

Disorders of brain development arise from a variety of causes (Aicardi, 1992; Capone, 1996; Nickel, 1992; Shonkoff & Marshall, 1990). Because brain formation is such a complex process, it is not surprising that it can be disturbed at any stage by numerous factors. Brain malformations may result from to genetic disorders, prenatal or perinatal insults, teratogens, metabolic insults, or infections. In as many as 60% of cases, brain abnormalities may have an obscure or unidentified etiology. These disorders may reflect a structural departure from normal brain development, and the functional and neuropsychological consequences can be extremely variable, ranging from severe disability to normal or near-normal function. Therefore, clinicians should not always assume the worst prognosis in such situations.

Malformation of the developing brain is a significant cause of severe mental retardation and developmental disability. Existing data suggest that 25% of conceptions are affected by a developmental CNS disturbance. Such disturbances account for a high percentage of fetal and infant deaths. This causative factor accounts for many "clinical" cases of mental retardation, in which the degree of limitation is severe and can occur regardless of environmental influences, family history, or SES. In actuality, malformation of the developing brain causes the mental retardation distribution as a whole to have an unexpected bimodal form. Epidemiological studies have indicated that prenatal factors are of major etiological importance in these cases.

A *primary malformation* refers to an anomaly that results from disruption of normal developmental events, resulting in failure in formation of an anatomic structure. Conversely, a *secondary malformation* results from the breakdown of a previously formed structure because of a destructive event such as infection or injury. Our understanding of malformations and ability to specify the nature and extent of an anomaly have expanded greatly with the introduction of procedures such as computerized tomography (CT) and magnetic resonance imaging (MRI). MRI is superior to the CT scan in diagnosing primary brain disorders (see Anderson & Gore, 1997).

The purpose of this discussion is to familiarize the clinician with brain disorders that may be encountered in the practice of infant and early childhood neuropsychology. These disorders place infants and young children at established and/or biological risks (Chapter 2). However, a detailed description of these brain disorders, or an all-inclusive listing, is beyond the scope of this text. Disorders of brain development will be divided into the following sections: (1) early brain malformations, (2) perinatal insults, (3) infections, and (4) other teratogens. Within each section, more common disorders will be described in an overview format to provide the clinician with a basic understanding of these disorders.

EARLY BRAIN MALFORMATIONS

Case 1. J. J. is an 18-month-old boy who was born with myelomeningocele. At 12 months his Bayley Scales of Infant Development-II Mental Developmental Index (MDI) was 106 (normal) and his Psychomotor Index (PDI) was 74 (borderline). He is returning for a follow-up neurodevelopmental evaluation. J. J.'s parents indicate that he has the ability to stand with support, but his fine motor skills are weak. They still don't understand what is causing his problem or what the prognosis might be, and are posing these questions to the developmental neuropsychologist.

Early brain malformations are frequently associated with genetic disorders, although etiologies often cannot be identified. The aforementioned stages of brain development and their associated malformations will be discussed below (see Chapter 3). Figure 4.1 is provided for reference; it depicts time lines for neuroanatomical development (Giedd, 1997).

Dorsal Induction

Induction refers to the influence of one tissue on another so that the second tissue differentiates into a completely different tissue than the first (Nickel, 1992). Primary disturbances of dorsal induction result in defects of neural tube closure, producing infants and children with large heads or spinal cord defects. These defects typically are readily apparent. The following are the most common malformations.

Anencephaly

Anencephaly results from failure of the anterior (rostral) portion of the neural tube to close by approximately 24 days. Cerebral structures are severely affected, and portions of the frontal, parietal, and occipital bones are undeveloped,

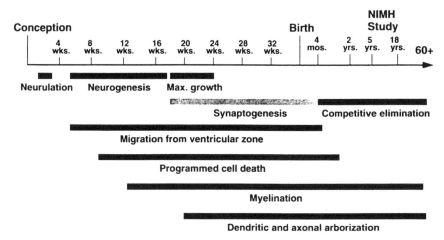

Figure 4.1. Time course of critical events in brain development. From J. N. Giedd, *Normal Development*, p. 269, 1997. Used with permission of W.B. Saunders Co.

creating a large opening in the skull. The exposed neural tissue has little resemblance to the normal structure of the brain. As this defect is usually incompatible with life, most early developmental neuropsychologists will not encounter infants with this disorder.

Encephalocele

This disorder is more restricted, and is the result of failure of a portion of the anterior area of the neural tube to close by day 26 of gestation. Most typically, the encephalocele occurs in the midline occipital region and less often in the midline frontal regions of the brain. The neural tissue protrudes through the bony defect and consists of cerebral cortex, white matter, and overlying meningeal membranes; other abnormalities of the cerebrum and cerebellum are common. Hydrocephalus often co-occurs, and surgical correction is often necessary. Neurodevelopmental outcome is variable, but mental retardation and severe motor deficits are common.

Myelomeningocele or Spina Bifida (Myelodysplasia)

Myelomeningocele is the most common anatomical malformation of the CNS. It results from the incomplete closure of the caudal portion of the neural tube and its coverings during the first month of pregnancy. Causes are multifactorial and include genetic and environmental factors. Associated factors include maternal diabetes, diet, use of valproate, and X-linked transmission (Welch & Lorenzo, 1991). The incidence of neural tube defects such as myelomeningocele is reduced by ingestion of folic acid supplements during early pregnancy.

In this condition, the skeletal and soft tissue coverings of a portion of the spinal cord do not develop; the spinal cord and nerves that exit the spinal canal at that location are abnormal ("dysplastic"), and are covered with only a thin membrane. The location determines the degree and type of neurodevelopmental dysfunction, with lower-level myelomeningocele having a better prognosis (80% are in the lumbar or lumbosacral region). This results in varying degrees of lower extremity motor impairment, sensory loss, and neurogenic bowel and bladder. Thoracic-region myelomeningocele usually results in severe curvature of the spine (kyphosis). Hydrocephalus eventually develops in 80%, and approximately 90% of children with myelomeningocele and hydrocephalus have the associated *Chiari malformation, Type II* (a malformation of the brain stem and cerebellum in which the medulla and cerebellum are displaced into the cervical canal).

Neuropsychological outcomes are variable, and a diagnosis of myelomeningocele does not necessarily have a poor outcome. Lesions above the L3 (lumbar) level result in complete loss of use of the lower extremities (paraplegia). With L3 and L4–L5 deformities, ambulation is possible with bracing and crutches. Associated anomalies, quality of medical care, shunt malfunctions requiring revisions, shunt infections, and environmental factors will affect the ultimate outcome. Ventriculitis is the most significant factor affecting cognitive outcome.

Hydrocephalus

This problem in commonly found with myelodysplasia (congenital), but also can arise from the consequences of perinatal problems (acquired). Cerebrospinal fluid (CSF) normally circulates through the ventricular system and then into the subarachnoid space where it nourishes the brain and spinal cord before it is reabsorbed. Interruption or obstruction in this circulation results in excessive volume of intracranial CSF with resultant fluid backup, increased pressure, and expansion of the ventricles. In hydrocephalus, the brain is under stress and there is deformation or compression in which liquid compartments intrude on the solid matter (Welch & Lorenzo, 1991). Surgical placement of a ventriculoperitoneal shunt is often necessary to drain fluid from the ventricles to the abdominal cavity.

Prolonged hydrocephalus can result in compression of the cerebral cortex which translates into neurodevelopmental morbidity; more than 50% of children with congenital hydrocephalus have mental retardation. Demyelination of the white matter often occurs and may explain why many individuals with hydrocephalus have poor fine motor skills (Sobkowiak, 1992). Spatial skills generally are less well developed relative to language skills. However, a so-called "cocktail party syndrome," may occur, which involves excessive verbalizing beyond that which the child actually comprehends. The presence of this syndrome is associated with mental deficiency. Again, shunt infections and malfunctions increase the likelihood of compromised outcomes.

Ventral Induction

Ventral induction involves the mesoderm at the rostral (head or cranial) end of the embryo. Disruptions in this process result in abnormalities of the face and brain. Essentially, the brain fails to cleave normally. Therefore, ventral induction disruption will affect the normal separation of the brain into two hemispheres.

Holoprosencephaly

Holoprosencephaly results from defective cleavage of the embryonic forebrain by the sixth week of gestation. The hallmark is severe midline dysgenesis (single-lobed brain) with fusion of structures such as the thalamus and basal ganglia, and absence of other structures such as the corpus callosum or septum. This disorder routinely is found in infants with certain genetic syndromes such as abnormalities in chromosomes 13 or 18. The *alobar* type is marked by severe facial deformities (eyes, nose) with accompanying brain anomalies. These children have poor developmental outcome, and die in infancy. The *lobar* type has differentiation of the third and lateral ventricles, and cleavage in the occipital lobe, but the anterior (front) section of the brain is fused. Microcephaly and severe to profound mental retardation with seizures are found frequently with this type. Occasionally, mild to moderate mental retardation without seizures has been reported.

Dandy Walker Malformation

Dandy Walker malformation is a related ventral induction disorder. It involves partial or complete agenesis of the cerebellar hemispheres (a cyst separates them) and is associated with hydrocephalus and other CNS abnormalities. More than 75% of these children have IQs less than 70, although often the mental retardation is related to the presence of other brain abnormalities.

Proliferation

Proliferation occurs during the second to fourth months of gestation. This stage is critical, because once neuronal proliferation stops, the final neuronal numbers are set. Disturbances result in too many or too few neurons being produced. Proliferation abnormalities typically affect the size of the head and the underlying cell development.

Microcephaly

Individuals with *micrencephaly* manifest *microcephaly*, defined as a head circumference smaller than 2 SDs below average (below the third centile) for the child's age and gender. These two terms technically are not synonymous. The term *micrencephaly* refers to a heterogeneous group of disorders characterized by reduced brain size and weight. Not all cases of micrencephaly represent a true disturbance of neuronal migration. Primary micrencephaly is usually associated with genetic or chromosomal abnormalities, major congenital anomaly/mental retardation syndromes, maternal toxic-metabolic disorders, or prenatal exposure to teratogens. In fact, more than 200 syndromes involve microcephaly. Secondary micrencephaly can be associated with primary disturbances of brain development such as holoprosencephaly or migrational disorder, or is secondary to an intrauterine or postnatal destructive lesion such as a vascular hypoxic ischemia. There is considerable variability in the degree of cognitive function attained by these children, ranging from normal levels to severe dysfunction. Generally, as development proceeds in infants and children with microcephaly, cognitive impairments become more evident. The etiology and associated abnormalities will influence the ultimate outcome. Head circumferences smaller than 3 SDs are more highly associated with mental retardation.

Megalencephaly

Megalencephaly refers to a heterogeneous group of disorders characterized by increased brain size and weight. Children with megalencephaly always manifest *macrocephaly*, defined as a head circumference 2–3 SDs above the mean. In *hypertrophy* of the brain, the enlarged brain size is the result of increased size of neural and glial elements, in *hyperplasia* there is an increased number of neurons and/or glia. Enlargement can be limited to the cerebral hemispheres or can include the entire brain. Again, the neuropsychological/neurodevelopmental outcomes vary, from severe (mental retardation, motor impairment, and seizures) to mild (learning disabilities, language problems, or minor neurological sequelae). There are familial forms of megalencephaly that are not routinely associated with neuropsychological problems.

Migration

Problems during this developmental phase can result in severe disruption of neuronal networks. The peak period of neuronal migration occurs between the third and fifth months of gestation. Disturbances in neuronal migration result in anomalous formation of the cortical plate and cortical columns. Diffuse distur-

bances produce cerebral palsy, learning disorders, or epilepsy; with focal disturbances, epilepsy is the main problem. Various types of epilepsy (e.g., infantile
spasms, other types of myoclonus) can result from dysplasias arising from
defects of neuronal migration (Gordon, 1996b). Migration disorders most likely
to be encountered by clinicians include the following.

Schizencephaly

This is a disorder of early neuronal migration (8 weeks), characterized by
complete agenesis of a section of the cerebral wall, resulting in a thickened
cortical mantle with deep seams or clefts. The cortex surrounding the cleft is
abnormal in terms of the actual cell structure or overall formations (e.g., gyri).
The outcome generally is poor (particularly when the clefts are bilateral), with
severe mental retardation, seizures, and neuromotor disorders such as hemiplegia
or quadriplegia being found (Gordon, 1996a).

Lissencephaly

This disorder also has an early occurrence (11–13 weeks) and is considered the
most severe neuronal migration disorder. It is characterized by agyria, i.e., absence
of secondary and tertiary gyri, which is manifested by a smooth brain surface.
Neuropsychological outcome is uniformly poor, with severe to profound mental
retardation, seizures, and motor dysfunctions. The severity of lissencephaly does
not necessarily correlate with the severity of clinical manifestations.

Pachygyria

This disorder is closely related to agyria and can coexist. Pachygyria is characterized by relatively few broad, flat, thick gyri, and few sulci. The cortical mantle
is thickened, and the cortex can contain four (versus the usual six) layers. The
sequelae are similar to lissencephaly, although perhaps somewhat less profound
(e.g., the infant may crawl, have some limited speech).

Polymicrogyria

Polymicrogyria has an onset no later than the fourth or fifth month of gestation.
The cortex contains a large number of very small gyri with shallow convolutions
(sulci). This condition gives the cortical surface a very wrinkled appearance,
sometimes likened to a "chestnut kernel" (Gordon, 1996a). The cortex is thick
and may contain a reduced number of layers. This disorder can be seen with
meningomyelocele and fetal cytomegalovirus exposure. If large sections of the

brain are affected, the child will have mental retardation, spasticity or hypotonia, and seizures. If the disorder is more focal, neuropsychological findings may be more limited, perhaps being evident only in terms of epilepsy.

Heterotopias

This disorder is considered a late neuronal migration disorder that occurs at 5–6 months gestation. The basic defect involves neuronal migration to abnormal locations, and the etiology can be genetic, chromosomal, or vascular. Some neurons may survive and form limited numbers of connections. Subependymal heterotopias cause bulging of the ventricular wall. Sometimes tiny herniations of neurons project from the cortical surface (brain warts). Although there have been reported associations with developmental language disorders, this type of neuronal migration disorder may also occur in apparently normal individuals. The nature and severity of neuropsychological symptoms most likely are dependent on the number, size, and location of these lesions.

Agenesis of the Corpus Callosum

This can occur early (11–12 weeks) or late (closer to 20 weeks). Early occurrence results in complete agenesis, whereas later occurrence causes partial agenesis. Essentially there is disruption in the corpus callosum, the white matter that connects both hemispheres. Outcomes vary and depend on the degree of agenesis, and the associated syndrome that may have caused the anomaly. Frequently there are developmental delays and seizures. In some series, however, as many as 15% of children with this disorder reportedly have normal intelligence. Seizures occurring in early infancy that result from agenesis of the corpus callosum have the worst prognosis.

Other disorders of late neuronal migration are caused by perinatal events such as subependymal hemorrhage or periventricular leukomalacia (discussed below). In these cases, the adverse event disrupts radial glial fibers (guides) that retract from the cortical surface, thereby preventing the cells from reaching their destinations. These stranded cells form collections of heterotopic gray matter. Impaired coordination, visual/perceptual problems and seizures often result.

Organization/Differentiation

A peak period for neural organization is difficult to determine, although the most rapid development in the cortex is between 6 months and postnatal year 2 or 3 (see Fig. 4.1). Genetic programming is substantial, but environmental influences are also important. Unfortunately, primary disturbances in brain organization and differentiation are not well understood. Disorders fall into one of the following categories: (1) axon/dendritic damage caused by infections or metabolic disorders, (2) synaptic loss related to intoxicants, (3) synaptic aberrance resulting from systemic disease, or (4) tissue infarction produced by maternal disease. Thus, the two main themes are disruptions in neuronal differentiation or in the development of synapses. The generalized, principal deficit in these disorders is reflected in aberrant cortical circuitry, which then alters the functional integrity of electrochemical signaling within the brain. Sequelae include sensory loss, motor loss, language deficit, speech deficit, or memory disorder. In individuals with mental retardation of an unidentified etiology, the organizational disturbances most consistently found are impaired dendritic arborization and poor development of the dendritic spines manifested by spine loss or preponderance of very long, thin, immature spines.

Myelination

Myelination occurs over a very prolonged period, beginning in the sixth month of gestation and proceeding into adulthood. Primary disturbances in myelination include cerebral white matter hypoplasia, amino acid defects, organic acid defects, degenerative diseases, and malnutrition.

Cerebral White Matter Hypoplasia

This condition is characterized by a marked deficiency in cerebral white matter. The nonprogressive clinical syndrome is manifested by spastic quadriplegia, seizures, and significant cognitive impairment. These symptoms are often apparent in the neonatal period.

Amino Acid Deficits

Phenylketonuria, nonketotic hyperglycinemia, and maple syrup urine disease are the most common amino acid disorders associated with problems in white matter production. By childhood, more severe reductions in myelin are present. Neurodevelopmental outcome is variable, and depends on whether specific therapies have been initiated (e.g., diet in the case of PKU).

Organic Acid Deficits

These disorders of metabolism produce similar neuropathological findings and progression of white matter lesions. They are characterized by the accumulation of compounds that cause acidosis. Referred to as *inborn errors of metabolism*, the problems are caused by abnormalities in vitamin metabolism, lipid metabolism, the citric acid cycle, and oxidative metabolism.

Degenerative Diseases

Neurodegenerative diseases that affect white matter are often genetically linked. Progressive loss of central white matter and interference with new myelin formation are hallmark characteristics, resulting in progressive loss of cognitive and motor skills and eventual death. Some examples of neurodegenerative diseases that clinicians may encounter include metachromatic leukodystrophy, adrenoleukodystrophy, and Krabbe disease. Neuromuscular disorders are diseases of the motor unit (anterior horn cell, its nerve fiber, and the muscle fibers that it innervates). Diseases of the anterior horn cell are called neuronopathies or motor neuron diseases. Diseases of the nerve are called neuropathies, disorders of the neuromuscular junction are referred to as myasthenia, and disorders of muscle are myopathies.

Malnutrition

Malnutrition early in infancy can also negatively affect brain development by causing decreased synthesis of myelin. This typically occurs postnatally, up through age 3 or 4. Increased risk for developmental sequelae exists, not only in terms of intelligence, but also for behavioral issues such as attention, activity, and social responsiveness.

PERINATAL INSULTS

Case 2. D. D. is a 12-month-old who was born at term gestational age (40 weeks). He currently shows weak tone of the upper extremities, tends to favor his left hand, and his verbal productions are minimal. D. D.'s 1-minute Apgar score was 5, and the question has been raised as to whether this was the "cause" of the infant's current problems.

Case 3. V. S. is a 6-month-old (corrected age) born at 28 weeks gestational age. She demonstrates increased tone of the lower extremities, tends to pull to stand versus sitting, and her parents have indicated that she had a "bleed" while in the neonatal intensive care unit. They are questioning the clinician as to how the current findings relate to V. S.'s perinatal course.

The spectrum of CNS disorders following perinatal insults is determined by the nature and severity of the insult, and by the brain's maturational stage at the time of insult (Hill & Volpe, 1989). Brain damage from severe *hypoxemia* (the reduction of oxygen in the blood) and *ischemia* (decreased blood flow to the brain) frequently produces permanent disabilities in infants and young children (Johnston, Trescher, & Taylor, 1995). Hypoxemia and ischemia are currently thought to trigger a *neurotoxic biochemical cascade* that produces permanent cell death over a period of hours to days. This cascade then causes synaptic dysfunction and overactivation of excitatory brain receptors. The effects differ, depending on gestational age: In premature infants, the periventricular white matter is especially vulnerable, whereas neuronal structures are more vulnerable at term and at later ages.

Much confusion arises regarding terminology used in discussion of the effects of perinatal events on infant and early childhood neuropsychology. Some of the major terms are defined in Table 4.1.

Perinatal asphyxia (*asphyxia neonatorum*) refers to disturbed exchange of oxygen and carbon dioxide caused by an interruption of respiration. Oxygen deficiency (*hypoxemia*) and carbon dioxide excess (*hypercarbia*) result in metabolic changes and a decrease in blood pH (*acidemia*). Decreased blood pressure and loss of autoregulation in the brain occur. Asphyxia may be prenatal, intrapartum (labor-related), or postnatal. In actuality, the term *asphyxia* is imprecise, because the intrapartum disruption of fetal blood flow is rarely, if ever, absolute. Although *perinatal asphyxia* and *hypoxic-ischemic encephalopathy* (HIE) are used interchangeably, the latter term actually refers to oxygen deprivation to the brain by the combined effects of hypoxemia and ischemia.

Table 4.1. Perinatal Insult Terminology

Term	Definition
Perinatal asphyxia	Disturbed exchange of oxygen and carbon dioxide; accompanied by multisystem organ dysfunction (cardiovascular, gastrointestinal, pulmonary, renal)
Hypoxic-ischemic encephalopathy (HIE)	Deprivation of oxygen to the brain due to the combined effects of hypoxemia and ischemia
Hypoxemia	Reduction of oxygen in the blood
Ischemia	Decreased blood flow to the brain
Cerebral palsy	Nonprogressive, motor disability, often evident from early infancy, although symptoms may vary somewhat over time
Acidemia	Profound acidemia is blood pH < 7.00
Anoxia	Complete lack of oxygen
Antepartum/antenatal period	Period from conception to onset of labor
Intrapartum period	Period from onset of labor to delivery
Neonatal period	Completion of delivery to 1 month of age

Asphyxia traditionally has been indexed as a low Apgar score (Apgar, 1953). The Apgar score is a rating of five objective signs scored at 1 and 5 minutes after birth. These signs (heart rate, respiratory effort, reflex irritability, muscle tone, and color) are rated 0–2, the maximum score being 10. (See Table 4.2.)

Although this is a quick method of assessing the state of the newborn infant, it has been misused in many outcome studies (American Academy of Pediatrics, 1996). Moreover, tone, color, and reflex irritability are dependent on the physiological maturity of the infant; as a result, preterm babies may receive a low score simply because of their gestational age. A low 1-minute Apgar score does not correlate with later outcome (AAP, 1996; Aylward, 1993). The 5-minute score may be more useful, particularly if *change* between 1 and 5 minutes is considered. However, even 5-minute scores of 0–3 have limited predictive utility, increasing the risk of cerebral palsy (CP) in term infants from 0.3% to approximately 1% (5-minute scores of 7–10 are considered normal and 4–6 intermediate). Predictive utility increases when the score remains in the 0–3 range at 10, 15, and 20 minutes, but even here some children will not demonstrate any neurodevelopmental sequelae (Freeman & Nelson, 1988). In fact, even if a full-term infant has an Apgar score of 0–3 at 5 minutes that improves to ≥ 4 at 10 minutes, there is at least a 90% chance of not having CP later. Conversely, 75% of children with CP have normal Apgar scores at birth. Therefore, Apgar scores should best be considered indicative of the infant's current condition only, and not a more long-term indicator of neuropsychological dysfunction. In fact, in 1867, Freud was a harbinger of this opinion, when he suggested that CP was most likely to result from events occurring earlier in pregnancy versus those that occur during the birth process.

A stronger relationship between biological variables such as asphyxia and later outcome has been reported in more contemporary samples (Aylward, 1993). In particular, the *types* of outcome measures that are employed may be critical.

Table 4.2. Apgar Scoring

Component	Score		
	0	1	2
Heart rate (beats/min)	Absent	Slow (<100)	>100
Respirations	Absent	Weak cry/ hypoventilation	Good, strong cry
Muscle tone	Limp	Some flexion	Active motion
Reflex irritability	No response	Grimace	Cry/active withdrawal
Color	Blue or pale	Body pink/ extremities blue	Completely pink

Source: Apgar, Holaday, James, Weisbrot, & Berrien (1958).

Besides more severe indicators such as CP, severe mental retardation, epilepsy, or sensory dysfunctions (where up to 65% of cases are the result of prenatal etiologies), more subtle, *high- prevalence/low-severity dysfunctions* (learning disabilities, attention-deficit hyperactivity disorders, behavior problems) need to be assessed. Moreover, arrays (versus individual) of initial, biological measures and those taken 6 hours later (e.g., pH) appear more indicative of change. Therefore, Apgar scores by themselves probably are not predictive; rather, change over time *may* indeed be. It has been suggested (AAP, 1996; Depp, 1995) that when one considers asphyxia, in addition to an Apgar score of 0–3 for longer than 5 minutes, the infant should also demonstrate: (1) profound acidemia (pH<7.00), (2) neurological manifestations (seizures, coma, hypotonia), and (3) multisystem organ dysfunction.

Hypoxic-Ischemic Encephalopathy (HIE)

As already indicated, although *asphyxia* and *perinatal HIE* are used interchangeably, it would be best to view asphyxia as the necessary, precipitating event for HIE. Perinatal HIE is the major determinant of neurodevelopmental morbidity and mortality in the neonatal period (Hill & Volpe, 1989), with 90% of cases originating before or during birth. Hypoxia and ischemia cause deficits in the brain's neuronal-synaptic machinery, and activate a receptor channel process that normally services important functions in learning, memory, and activity-dependent plasticity (Johnston et al., 1995). There are neuroanatomical and behavioral indicators that differ depending on the infant's gestational age. Therefore, HIE will be discussed separately for full-term and preterm infants.

HIE in Full-Term Infants

In full-term infants, asphyxia occurs in 2–4/1000 births, with mortality ensuing in 30%; 25% of the surviving infants have HIE. In full-terms, the parasagittal regions—the "watershed" zone of arterial blood supply to the brain—are affected. This area is between the anterior, middle, and posterior cerebral arteries. Selective neuronal necrosis (cell death) occurs in the cerebral cortex, diencephalon, brain stem, cerebellum, and spinal cord. Injury to the basal ganglia and thalamus occurs more frequently in the term than in the preterm infant. In addition to neuronal loss, abnormalities in myelination occur, with alterations in the amount of and abnormal distribution of myelinated fibers. There is also cell death in the parietal–occipital area and adjacent white matter. The severity, duration, and timing of the insult determine the magnitude of brain injury. Prolonged, partial hypoxia seems to result in more variable injury, including diffuse cerebral necrosis with relative sparing of the deep cerebral structures.

Less severe insult may result in injury principally involving the watershed zones (parasagittal regions). The stage of regional structural and biochemical development of the CNS appears to be a critical factor in determining HIE lesions. Areas of primary myelination, adjacent subcortical white matter, as well as the thalamus, basal ganglia, and brain stem are vulnerable. It is postulated that selective damage occurs in those areas that, at the moment of HIE insult, had achieved higher rates of oxygen–glucose utilization (Azzarelli, Caldemeyer, Phillips, & DeMeyer, 1996).

Clinical features of severe HIE in term newborns can include decreased level of consciousness, seizures (particularly "subtle seizures" involving abnormal ocular or facial movements), brain-stem dysfunction, motor abnormalities, and increased intracranial pressure. In less severe cases involving the area of the watershed zone corresponding to upper extremity function, there is weakness of the shoulder girdle and proximal upper extremities. Focal ischemic injury may present as unilateral weakness (hemiparesis). Classification of the spectrum of HIE correlates with long-term outcome, with severity being *mild, moderate*, or *severe* (Table 4.3). There is a high incidence of long-term neuropsychological sequelae if moderate or severe encephalopathy persists for longer than 7 days. Seizures related to HIE typically occur at 12–24 hours of age and may be transient or protracted.

HIE in Preterm Infants

HIE in the preterm infant is characterized by periventricular leukomalacia (PVL), selective neuronal necrosis, multifocal ischemic cerebral necrosis, and periventricular hemorrhagic infarction (PVI). Neuronal injury may be more prominent in the thalamus, brain stem, hippocampus, germinal matrix, and periventricular white matter, with relative sparing of the cerebral cortex. As a result, this type of damage often produces some degree of spasticity and resultant motor problems, and high-prevalence/low-severity dysfunctions. Lower ex-

Table 4.3. Behavioral Correlates of HIE

Mild	Hyperalertness, uninhibited reflexes, irritability, jitteriness, sympathetic overactivity, duration < 24 hours, not associated with long-term sequelae
Moderate	Lethargy, stupor, hypotonia, decrease in or suppressed primitive reflexes, seizures, decrease in spontaneous movements; 20–40% have neuropsychological sequelae, particularly if moderate HIE persists > 1 week
Severe	Coma, flaccid tone, suppressed brain-stem function, seizures, increased intracranial pressure; virtually all survivors have major neurodevelopmental sequelae (microcephaly, mental retardation, cerebral palsy, epilepsy)

Source: Adapted from Hill & Volpe (1989), Robertson & Finer (1985), Sarnat & Sarnat (1976).

tremities routinely are more affected than upper ones because of the proximity of lower extremity neuronal fibers of the watershed zone to the more vulnerable area. In contrast to term infants, where the concentrated neuronal circuits in the cerebral cortex and basal ganglia are predisposed to injury, preterm infants are more vulnerable to damage in the developing white matter. The two major disorders in preterm infants that result from HIE are PVL and PVI.

PVL is necrosis (cell death) of the white matter behind and to the side of the lateral ventricles. There is glial and neuronal loss, and cystic cavities (porencephalic) may develop, giving the brain a "Swiss cheese" look. With less severe degrees of damage, there is decreased cerebral myelination. Because of the rich arterial microvascular network in the area surrounding the ventricles, less ischemia is needed to cause damage at younger gestational ages. Rapid fluctuations in arterial blood pressure, and decreased blood flow exacerbate the vulnerability of actively differentiating and myelinating periventricular glial cells (Volpe, 1992). PVL can cause spastic diplegia (spasticity of the legs) or spastic quadriplegia (involving all four extremities). Visual and auditory impairment may also occur. The highest incidence of PVL occurs in infants born at 27–30 weeks gestation, with a peak at 28 weeks; infection and premature rupture of the membranes have been indicated as two major risk factors for PVL (particularly in combination) (Zupan et al., 1996).

PVI is hemorrhagic cell death (necrosis) of periventricular white matter that is large and asymmetric, frequently occurring with Grade IV intraventricular hemorrhage (approximately 15% of infants with severe IVH display this problem). Grade I and II IVH (see below) appear to arise primarily from fluctuation in blood flow within the immature brain vasculature, and less often result from HIE (Johnston et al., 1995). In more than two-thirds of cases of PVI, the lesions are unilateral, occurring in the periventricular white matter of the frontal-parieto-occipital regions. Even if the lesions are bilateral, they are asymmetric. Extensive infarctions are associated with high mortality rates, with localized infarctions having a better prognosis. Often a blood clot from the IVH causes obstruction of terminal veins. Upper and lower extremity involvement occurs, because the lesion affects descending motor fibers. The asymmetry can cause spastic hemiparesis or asymmetric quadriparesis and variable intellectual deficits.

Clinical features associated with cerebral injury in preterm infants include irritability, hypertonia of the lower extremities, increased neck extensor tone, apnea, poor feeding and clinical seizures (10–30% of cases) (Roland & Hill, 1995).

Periventricular/intraventricular hemorrhage (PVH/IVH) is characteristic of preterm infants <32 weeks gestational age, with an incidence of 35–45% (Volpe, 1987). It involves bleeding into the subependymal germinal matrix to varying degrees. Because this is the area where cell proliferation occurs, there is a high degree of vascularization. Obstructive hydrocephalus is a frequent

Table 4.4. Grading of Severity of Periventricular-Intraventricular Hemorrhage

Grade I	Subependymal/germinal matrix hemorrhage with no or minimal IVH (<10% of ventricular area). *Mild.*
Grade II	Intraventricular hemorrhage (10–50% of ventricular area). No ventricular dilatation. *Moderate.*
Grade III	Intraventricular hemorrhage (>50% of ventricular area: usually distends lateral ventricle). *Severe.*
Grade IV	Hemorrhagic intracerebral involvement or other parenchymal lesion, with 60% mortality rate. *Severe + intracerebral involvement.*

Source: Adapted from Papile, Burstein, Burnstein, & Koffler (1978), Volpe (1987).

complication. Fluctuating cerebral blood flow, increase in cerebral blood flow, increase in venous pressure, decrease in cerebral blood flow, and asphyxia (all the result of problems frequently found in preterm infants) may cause PVH/IVH. Cranial ultrasound scans are used to document IVH, and a typical grading scheme is shown in Table 4.4. In general, fewer neurodevelopmental problems are found with Grade I (5–10%) and Grade II (15–20%) IVH, and the incidence of problems increases with Grade III (35–50%) IVH. These deficits typically involve motor function, but if the bleeding extends into the adjacent cerebral white matter, the extent and severity of disabilities increase. However, more recently, increased risk of disability at preschool and school age has been reported for children who had Grade I and II hemorrhages (Lowe & Papile, 1990; van de Bor et al., 1993). Therefore, children with milder bleeds still are at risk for later problems. PVH/IVH occurs most commonly during the first 72 hours after birth, and small preterm infants (<1000 g) are predisposed to earlier bleeding than their heavier counterparts. Early ventriculomegaly (dilatation of the ventricles) is associated with neurodevelopmental problems.

Grade IV involves the presence of parenchymal blood, and as already indicated, probably does not reflect extension of ventricular bleeding, but rather is related to hemorrhagic infarction. Therefore, although Grades I–III may be considered to be on a continuum, Grade IV reflects a discrete event (even though it follows smaller bleeds). Ninety percent of survivors will have significant neurodevelopmental sequelae.

INFECTIONS OF THE CNS

Case 4. L. K. is a 10-year-old who was diagnosed with *Haemophilus influenzae* type b infection at the age of 9 months. He currently is demonstrating problems with attention and with reading comprehension. His physician recently called the developmental neuropsychologist to see if there might be a connection between L. K.'s early illness and his current problems.

Acute or chronic infections of brain tissue (*encephalitis*) or the meninges (membrane covering the brain; *meningitis*) cause significant neuropsychological impairment. During the prenatal period, a variety of congenital infections are known to cause neurodevelopmental disorders. Meningitis and encephalitis are postnatal disorders that produce a wide range of sequelae. These infections are associated with a variety of neuropsychological outcomes, ranging from minimal damage and normal function to major insult and severe disability. The brain injury can be static (nonprogressive), or it can be more insidious, with a gradual appearance of deficits. Some deficits may not emerge until later in infancy or early childhood (e.g., CP). The timing of infection and the infant's individual susceptibility are critical factors.

Toxoplasmosis

Congenital toxoplasmosis is caused by a protozoan parasite, often introduced by cats as the host. The mothers are asymptomatic, and transfer the parasite to their fetus, usually after the second month of gestation. Approximately 10% of infants are symptomatic in the newborn period; resultant problems include prematurity, microcephaly, hydrocephalus, seizures, CNS calcifications, and chorioretinitis (damage to the eyes). However, most infants are initially asymptomatic, with the most common problem being chorioretinitis, which can result in unilateral or bilateral blindness. Intellectual deficits may also be present, although emergence of these deficits may be delayed. Anatomically, cerebral lesions, necrosis, and obstruction of CSF flow (with resulting hydrocephalus) occur. The destructive lesions may be extensive.

Cytomegalovirus (CMV)

CMV is the most common viral disease transmitted in utero that negatively affects neuropsychological functioning. The frequency in the United States is approximately 1%, and the transmission rate from an infected mother is 24%. Intrauterine growth retardation (IUGR), microcephaly, seizures, mental retardation, prematurity, retinal problems, hearing loss, and meningoencephalitis occur, particularly if the infant demonstrates symptoms at birth. More than 90% of infected babies are asymptomatic at birth and these children have a better prognosis, although hearing and learning problems frequently occur. The virus has an affinity for rapidly growing germinal cells of the lateral ventricles, leading to periventricular lesions, necrosis, and calcifications. Polymicrogyria may also occur.

Rubella

Congenital rubella is characterized by IUGR, cataracts and other eye problems (retinitis), microcephaly, and heart and other organ involvement. Approximately 25% have neurological symptoms at birth (microcephaly, lethargy, irritability, hypotonia); 33–40% display psychomotor retardation by the end of the first year of life. Progressive visual and hearing deficits often occur. Timing of infection is critical, with severe CNS malformations occurring if the virus is introduced before week 12 of gestation; deafness alone occurs if it is introduced at 13–16 weeks of gestation. Rubella in the second trimester is associated with delayed mental development and communication skills, and decreased brain weight (of approximately 25%). It appears that inhibition of cell proliferation and meningeal or brain lesions occur. Autistic and other behavior disorders are associated with rubella as well. Some children exposed to rubella are asymptomatic, especially if they are infected later in pregnancy.

Herpes Simplex Virus (HSV)

Most cases of HSV infection with neuropsychological sequelae are related to HSV type 2. The fetus is at risk in the first half of pregnancy (first 20 weeks) and at birth, particularly the latter. There is a high incidence of spontaneous abortions and stillbirths. Encephalitis-type disease usually presents at 15–17 days, with seizures, irritability, poor feeding, bulging fontanelle, and pyramidal tract signs. Severe brain abnormalities can occur, including microcephaly, hydranencephaly, cysts, and mental retardation.

Human Immunodeficiency Virus (HIV)

HIV infection is transmitted to the fetus in approximately 30% of cases, with the infection occurring in the pre-, peri-, and postnatal periods. Vertical transmission (i.e., the infection is passed perinatally from mother to child) accounts for the largest number of new cases. Encephalopathy and other infections occur, with many infants dying by 12–18 months. Survival time after diagnosis appears to depend on a number of factors, including the timing of infection during gestation, premature birth, nutritional status, route of transmission, and type of other acquired infectious agents (e.g., CMV) (Johnson, 1993). Bacterial, viral, and fungal infections are part of the disease spectrum in children with HIV, including and resulting in lymphocytic interstitial pneumonitis (lung infection), failure to thrive, chronic diarrhea, and intractable thrush. The neuropsychological presentation in children is variable and may include developmental delay, motor impairment, and encephalopathy. The term *HIV encephalopathy* or *neuroaids* is used to refer to children with delayed motor and/or mental milestones, abnormal motor signs, weakness, disordered brainstem function, ataxia, blindness, secondary microcephaly, and seizures (Diamond & Cohen, 1992). Autopsy studies have revealed decreased brain weight, and calcifications of the vascular system in the region of the basal ganglia and deep cerebral white matter. The thalamus and brain stem are often affected as well. Three patterns of neurodevelopmental decline appear to emerge: (1) infants who demonstrate symptoms very early, with a progressive decline and relentless loss of developmental milestones, including those involving motor, social, and language skills, spasticity, and acquired microcephaly, (2) those who develop neuropsychological deterioration in early childhood or school age, with academic and attentional difficulties as markers of a declining course, and (3) children who display a more subacute course, interrupted by plateaus, milestone acquisition being initially slow followed by protracted plateau without further, new acquired skills, and accompanied by mild spasticity. In the young child, developmental sequelae include impaired brain growth, *progressive* motor dysfunction, motor delays, increasing spasticity (particularly of the lower extremities), delays or regression in social smile, delays or regression in vocalization/speech, and generalized developmental delay. In older children, sequelae include psychomotor slowing, emotional lability, social withdrawal, attentional difficulties, and visual-spatial/visual-perceptual dysfunction (Johnson, 1993). The neurodevelopmental course is affected by pharmacological treatment including AZT, DDI (dideoxyinosine), and DDC (dideoxycytidine), although no clear patterns have emerged regarding the effects of treatment on cognitive functioning. Presently, it is not clear if CNS disease results from direct or indirect effects of HIV infection to the brain (or both), but the end result is cerebral devastation (Mintz, 1996).

Haemophilus influenzae Type b

Other infections such as *H. influenzae* type b (Hib meningitis) may also cause CNS damage later in infancy. This disorder is the most common form of bacterial infection of meningeal tissues, which results in vascular inflammation, vessel occlusion, cerebral edema, hydrocephalus, and subdural effusions. Ischemia and direct compression of the brain are the primary causes of damage (Taylor, Schatschneider, & Rich, 1992). Hib meningitis occurs in 30 to 70 out of 100,000 children with 99% of cases before 5 years of age (most are in infancy). Sequelae include mental retardation (2–17%), hearing loss (10%), seizures (30%), hemiparesis/motor dysfunction (2–7%), and frequent learning disorders, with PIQs being lower than VIQs (Taylor et al., 1992).

OTHER TERATOGENS AFFECTING THE CNS

> **Case 5.** L.T., age 2 months, has been put up for adoption. She reportedly was exposed in utero to cocaine. She shows no physical abnormalities, and the prospective adoptive parents would like the clinician to evaluate the infant and discuss with them the potential effects cocaine exposure might have on L.T. as she gets older.

A variety of drugs can disrupt the development and function of the CNS in fetuses and infants. Unfortunately, there are serious methodological problems in the existing literature on drug effects and specific outcomes, thereby precluding the identification of a direct cause–effect relationship (e.g., Aylward, 1982; Mayes, Granger, Bornstein, & Zuckerman, 1992). Small subject numbers, lack of control for confounding variables (e.g., environmental issues, see Chapter 2), polydrug usage, and weak outcome measures all contribute to this confusion. Nonetheless, some generalizations can be made.

Cocaine Hydrochloride

Cocaine hydrochloride readily crosses the placenta and affects nerve endings and chemical messenger transmission. Fetal injury from maternal cocaine ingestion can take place directly and indirectly. Indirect injury occurs as a result of drug effects on maternal physiology. Direct effects involve the influence of the drug on fetal and peripheral nervous system development. With prolonged exposure to cocaine, dopamine depletion occurs, which can adversely affect the developmental outcome of the child exposed in utero to cocaine. Other physiological changes include a marked rise in maternal and fetal systolic blood pressure, reduction in uterine blood flow, and decreased fetal oxygenation. The concentration in the brain may be as much as 20 times higher than in plasma. Cocaine can therefore affect the regions of the brain crucial for learning, memory, behavioral, and cognitive functions (Phillips, Sharma, Premachandra, Vaughn, & Reyes-Lee, 1996). Investigations of neurological status of cocaine-exposed infants during the neonatal period have suggested many possible atypical features. These include: an increase in abnormal responses on the Neonatal Behavioral Assessment Scale (Brazelton, 1973), abnormalities in cry, abnormal sensorineural activity, an increase in CNS structural lesions (including hemorrhage), an increase in irritability, with poor state modulation, reduced self-quieting activity, and tone and movement abnormalities (Hurt et al., 1995). However, these findings are often conflicting. Problems with early state regulation (particularly self-quieting, lability, and irritability), habituation, and later attention and behavior problems (arousal, emotional control) have been reported more consistently (e.g., Phillips et al., 1996). Lower developmental and intelligence scores are not found as consistently, but there is a definite trend toward lower scores in cocaine-exposed infants. The mechanism of the teratogenic effects of cocaine is unclear, although the destructive neural effects may be secondary to the drug's vasoactive effect. Microcephaly, agenesis of the corpus callosum, hydrocephalus, and schizencephaly have been reported, and undoubtedly, the different types of abnormalities reflect differences in timing, amount, and duration of drug exposure. Infarctions in the frontal white matter, basal ganglia, and germinal matrix have also been reported.

Alcohol

Ethanol exposure can lead to fetal alcohol syndrome (FAS) or more subtle fetal alcohol effects (FAE). Thus, the effects of prenatal alcohol exposure should be considered to occur on a continuum, with FAE occurring more than twice as frequently as FAS. Ethanol exposure may affect all organ systems and may induce fetal hypoxia. The diagnosis of FAS is made when a recognizable pattern of malformation is noted, which includes specific facial abnormalities, somatic growth failure, and organic brain dysfunction. The typical facial abnormalities are found in a "T"-shaped area of the central facial region; these include short palpebral fissures (small eyes), epicanthal folds, premaxillary overgrowth with resultant flat, smooth philtrum, thin upper lip, and flattening of the medial midface. Failure of somatic growth is often seen, with height less than the 10th percentile for age and frequent failure to thrive (light weight for height). Brain involvement is manifested by microcephaly and behavioral/cognitive deficits including learning disabilities, perceptual problems, mild mental retardation, delayed adaptive behavior, ADHD, and behavior problems. In infancy, 75% show irritability, tremulousness, difficulties with sucking, and poor muscle tone (hypotonia). Again, the amount, duration, timing, and use of other drugs in conjunction with alcohol will determine the type and severity of neuropsychological dysfunction. Neuropathological findings include excessive neuronal migration and heterotopias, and dendritic spine abnormalities. Ethanol affects many aspects of neuronal development, including cell proliferation, migration, synaptogenesis, myelination, and neurotransmitter function. Abnormalities in glial cell development or function may represent a common underlying mechanism for these effects. The hippocampus and cerebellum are particularly sensitive to ethanol-induced damage.

Other Drugs

Some antiepileptic drugs (phenytoin, barbiturates, carbamazepine, sodium valproate) can cause CNS malformations, IUGR, and later behavioral and cognitive changes (Yerbi, 1988). Narcotics (heroin, codeine, methadone) produce fetal growth retardation, premature birth, withdrawal symptoms, and a small head. Infants exposed to phencyclidine (PCP) often initially are hypertonic and jittery, and later have problems in fine motor movements.

Polychlorinated Biphenyls, Dioxins, and Dibenzofurans

Polychlorinated biphenyls (PCBs), dioxins (polychlorinated dibenzo-p-dioxins; PCDDs), and dibenzofurans (PCDFs) are widespread, potentially neurotoxic environmental contaminants. Perinatal exposure occurs prenatally via the placenta, and postnatally via breast milk. Higher levels of these toxins in breast milk have been associated with reduced neonatal neurological optimality, and a higher incidence of neonatal hypotonia. These findings suggest neurotoxic effects of these compounds on the developing brain of neonates and the need for long-term follow-up (Huisman et al., 1995).

Conclusions

Studies of infants exposed in utero to various drugs present a spectrum of findings beginning with no apparent effects to significant neuropsychological impairment. Timing of drug usage during fetal life, type of drug, amount of usage (constant, occasional, binges), duration, individual vulnerability, and concomitant risk factors (polydrug use, nutrition, other environmental factors), and caregiving competence all will influence outcome. Therefore, the multifactorial nature of these influences results in penetrance of injury that is not uniform, with the influence being both subtle and complicated. It is unlikely that a dose–response curve will be established in this regard. Moreover, a period of neurobehavioral recovery and reorganization follows in the weeks to months after birth for many of these children.

SUMMARY

Brain injury in infants and young children can be caused by a variety of factors including: genetic disturbances, trauma, hemorrhage, stroke, infection, metabolic changes, lack of oxygen, and toxins. Each directly and indirectly destroys some portion of the brain, or prevents normal development and maturation. In aggregrate, there are a very large number of potential problems of a subtle nature as well (Lenn, 1991). Subtle metabolic and chemical changes occur, which may add to the insult, cause the dysfunction, and/or interfere with recovery. Some changes may actually promote recovery. These issues may explain why neuropsychological deficits are variable in infants and children with the same apparent CNS insult. Moreover, fetuses and infants are especially vulnerable to damage because of their reduced blood–brain barrier (designed to prevent chemicals from entering the brain); an early injury or defect may then affect the entire sequence of development that follows.

Early maternal malnutrition (particularly lack of essential fatty acids, vitamin E, and trace elements) leads to a reduction of total cell numbers and synapse formation, and may also interfere with neuronal migration. In addition, at 26–34 weeks gestation (when most premature infants are born), the normal process of neuron loss and axon retraction is at its height, with increased metabolic activity (and, hence, vulnerability). This increased activity is particularly located around the areas of the basal ganglia, caudate nucleus, cerebellum, and optic radiations—areas critical to motor control. These same areas are vulnerable to hemorrhage, ischemia, and disturbances of cerebral blood flow. Periventricular hemorrhage also leads to impaired myelination. Thus, perinatal insult will result in disturbances of synapse formation, development of neuronal connections to the cerebral cortex, and postnatal myelination. In addition to white matter damage, diffuse damage to the gray matter, particularly in the area of the hippocampus (involved in the translation of shorter-term to long-term memory) and the cerebellum, has been found in preterm infants born at 28–32 weeks gestation (e.g., Mutch, Leyland, & McGee, 1993; Volpe, 1987).

With respect to *neuroplasticity*, the effects of CNS damage depend on where the insult occurs, and at what age. Three major systems are known to exhibit plasticity in response to brain injury: visual, motor, and language (Lenn, 1991). Plasticity is in terms of structure-function relationships, at the synaptic level. If the damage is too severe, or if structures are absent or malformed (as in the case of early brain malformations), the degree of neuroplasticity is severely limited. Plasticity also is dependent on the fact that brain activity can be considered on two time scales: *moment to moment*, and *longer term* (Lenn, 1991). Moment-to-moment changes involve "automatic" reactions that do not require special attention and without memory formation of the event. These changes in the brain are mostly electrical, with instantaneous changes in the size and shape of existing synapses and complex chemical events that last for only milliseconds (e.g., an infant reacts to light). Longer-term changes involve the incorporation of attention, which strengthens and retains synapses (e.g., the infant pays attention to a pattern of light while lying in a crib). Although vision is the same whether the infant pays attention or not, the difference is in whether synapses emanating from the attention center are active while the infant gazes at the pattern. If both types of synapses are active at the same time, more synaptic "glue" is produced by the dendrite at the site of the active synapses; the more "glue," the greater the likelihood that the synapse will be retained. Therefore, synapses are made and modified during normal development and learning. Damage can eradicate neurons, axons, and synaptic formations. If connections are made between damaged cells and distant undamaged cells, additional events could occur; this depends on whether the undamaged cells send axons to the damaged area or receive input (via synapses) from the damaged area. In the former, cells will survive if they have other connections to undamaged areas by forming new synapses with surviving nerve cells. In the latter, distant undamaged cells that have lost input from the damaged area may attract sprouts from nearby axons and form synapses. However, such changes are not always positive. Therefore, it becomes apparent how different types of CNS insults, the system involved, and the timing of insult can affect such connections. For example, in the motor system, there appears to be both a critical period that ends at term birth during which normal synapse elimination is reduced to compensate for injury, and a period from birth to 1 year of age when partial compensation occurs (Lenn, 1991).

This discussion relates to that at the end of the previous chapter; the key issue is that integration of functional units of the brain is critical to efficient neuropsychological operations. Those processes that are repeated and that involve integration of different units (as in the case of attention and visual input) are critical to higher-order processes of learning and memory. However, almost paradoxically, these integrated units may be more sensitive to CNS insult, yet at the same time be more likely to recover, because of neuroplasticity. Moreover, these units and their integration may shed light on development of the high-prevalence/low-severity dysfunctions such as learning and attention disorders. This fact has important ramifications in terms of the neuropsychological/neurodevelopmental assessment of infants and young children, as discussed in the next chapter.

Assessment

Recently, Capute and Accardo (1996) stated that "developmental pediatrics is the closest approximation to a neuropsychology of childhood" (p. 22). This statement again underscores the considerable overlap between developmental assessment and infant and early childhood neuropsychology. These authors also acknowledge that the models of brain function used in assessment of adults do not apply to infancy or early childhood. In this young population, the diagnosis of CNS impairment is routinely made on the basis of deviations from a normal pattern of milestone achievement, and the deviance in behavior can be quantitative or qualitative. The latter point is important, because many developmental assessment instruments that are used to evaluate infants and young children rely solely on quantitative information, and disregard *how* the infant or young child achieves a score. There are many ways in which an endpoint milestone such as walking or placing small beads in a box may be achieved. The method and quality of milestone achievement (i.e., "ways") are equally if not more important than whether the test item is passed. Stated differently, in early developmental neuropsychology, a child's developmental pattern cannot simply be reduced to or summarized by a single number or score.

DELAY, DISSOCIATION, AND DEVIANCE

Related to the evaluation of developmental problems are the concepts of delay, dissociation, and deviance (Capute & Accardo, 1996). A delay occurs when a child does not reach developmental milestones at the expected age, allowing for the broad variation of "normality." The lag could occur in one or more areas of neurodevelopmental function. A delay per se is not intrinsically abnormal. However, inherent in the concept is the supposition that the infant or child will "catch up." Therefore, *delay* cannot be used indefinitely. A dissociation refers to a difference between developmental rates of two "streams" or areas of development. A major discrepancy between receptive and expressive language abilities, or verbal versus visual processing would be considered dissociations.

A dissociation could also occur if two typically related or linked neurodevelopmental acquisitions did not occur together, as in the case of an infant who crawls but does not sit unsupported. A child with cerebral palsy (CP) may be able to roll over at a precocious age (because of increased tone), but not be able to pull-to-sit. Again, a dissociation is not necessarily abnormal, although there is an increased likelihood of such. *Deviance* is a nonsequential unevenness in the achievement of "milestones" or the appearance of an atypical developmental indicator, and is *abnormal* at any age. Significant hypertonicity of the lower extremities, cortical thumbing, or the infant who pulls to stand in the pull to sit maneuver are examples of deviance.

EVALUATION MATRIX

This discussion is elaborated in the evaluation matrix of Fig. 5.1, where five areas are considered: (1) the results of the neurodevelopmental screen/assessment, (2) the environment, (3) the actual area of function that is assessed, (4) the age of the child, and (5) the medical and developmental history. All five areas work in a dynamic fashion. In the clinical reasoning process the importance of each of these five areas must be weighed and their interrelationships considered, in order to accurately determine the importance and prognostic value of specific findings.

Developmental Screen/Assessment Results

The actual test or evaluation instrument is important, as is its reliability, validity, sensitivity, and specificity. Without going into psychometric theory in detail, the test data should be reproducible, able to be obtained consistently and by different examiners (reliability), and the test should measure what it is supposed to measure (validity). *Sensitivity* refers to the test accurately identifying an infant or child as

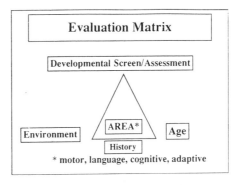

Figure 5.1. Evaluation matrix.

"not normal" when he or she actually has a neurodevelopmental problem; *specificity* requires that a normal child be identified as "normal" by the test. Unfortunately, in infant and early childhood neuropsychology, there is no "gold standard." As a result, *co-positivity* and *co-negativity* are often used in place of *sensitivity* and *specificity*, respectively. *Relative risk* or odds ratios are often recommended for use in early developmental neuropsychology, because they provide estimates (including confidence intervals) of the likelihood of having or not having later problems, based on findings of an earlier neuropsychological assessment. For example, a child receiving an "abnormal" evaluation at age 6 months might be five times more likely to have an "abnormal" neuropsychological evaluation at 3 years of age than a child who had a "normal" evaluation at 6 months.

Moreover, a critical concept in developmental neuropsychology is *age-related manifestations*, where certain skills (or deficits) become more visible as the child grows. Neuropsychological problems can be "dormant" or silent until the function affected by the particular deficit is involved in a specific test behavior or developmental acquisition. This may explain why the prevalence of disabilities increases with age, being approximately 1–2% from 0 to 24 months and rising to 8% at 24 to 60 months. In reference to actual evaluation results, the degree or magnitude of dysfunction also must be considered, particularly in terms of prognosis and intervention.

Environment

This aspect of the evaluation matrix was addressed in Chapter 2. Certain areas of development (e.g., language) are more affected by environment than others (e.g., expressive motor). In addition, environmental influences vary depending on the child's age; for example, the influences are much more noticeable from approximately 18 to 24 months and upwards. The effects of intervention programs also must be considered in this area. The clinician should therefore factor in environmental considerations in early neuropsychological assessment, as these would affect interpretation of test findings and their implications, particularly in terms of intervention.

Area of Function

In infant and early childhood neuropsychology, areas of function include Neurological Functions/Intactness, Receptive Functions (visual, auditory, verbal), Expressive Functions (gross motor, fine motor, oral-motor, verbal), and Cognitive Processes (problem solving, object permanency, imitation, goal-directedness, mental activity) (Aylward, 1995) (see Chapter 1). This organizational framework differs slightly from areas or streams of development frequently cited in the developmental literature, namely, Motor (gross, fine), Language (receptive, expressive, articulation), Cognitive, and Adaptive/Personal-Social. Nonetheless, the two schemas are conceptually similar. In general, language and cognitive areas are much better predictors of later intelligence than are motor or adaptive/personal-social areas. Language deficits become more obvious with increasing age, whereas there is a tendency for mild and moderate neuromotor dysfunction to improve as the child grows older.

Age

The age at time of evaluation is important for several reasons. First, the natural course of certain neuropsychological problems may improve or worsen with increasing age (as in the case of motor versus language function). Second, certain functions emerge at later ages, and therefore are more likely to be evaluated accurately (cognitive processes). Results of earlier evaluations also can be compared with those obtained later to determine consistency of findings.

Related to age is the issue of correction for prematurity in the case of infants born prior to term gestational age. Correction for prematurity involves subtracting the number of weeks that the infant was born prior to term (40 weeks gestational age) from the child's chronological age. Therefore, a child born prematurely at 28 weeks gestational age and evaluated at 9 months chronological age will have a corrected or conceptional age of 6 months. Although there continues to be debate regarding whether or not to correct, the general consensus is that correction is necessary (Blasco, 1989; Lems, Hopkins, & Samsom, 1993; Miller, Dubowitz, & Palmer, 1984). What remains to be clarified, however, is the degree of correction and the time frame over which it is employed. It appears that full correction is necessary over the first year, but there is no well-grounded consensus regarding correction between 12 and 24 months. Many infant tests (e.g., BINS; Aylward, 1995) endorse correction up to and including 2 years of age. Ultimately, an algorithm is needed that would include the infant's gestational age, age at time of testing, and area that is being assessed. Such an algorithm would consider all three factors and produce a graduated correction formula. Until such a procedure is developed, it appears best to correct fully for prematurity until 2 years of age. However, the clinician should also consider both corrected and noncorrected scores. Obviously, no problem occurs if the uncorrected score is in the "optimal" or "normal" range. Similarly, if a corrected score falls in the "nonoptimal" or "abnormal" range, definite concern is warranted. The situation is not as clear-cut when the diagnosis would differ depending on which scoring strategy is employed. The situation is compounded by inaccuracy inherent in estimation of gestational age, and lack of consensus as to whether to correct to 40 weeks or 37 weeks (definition of full-term gestation endorsed by the World Health Organization). This latter issue would be particularly important in the case of a 36-week-old infant where correction could be either 1 or 4 weeks.

The congruence between events occurring in the child's medical history and neuropsychological findings offers additional evaluation information (see Chapter 4). For example, severe HIE places a child at significant risk for cognitive and motor deficits, whereas Grade III IVH potentially has a more significant impact on motor function. Consideration of the type of neuropsychological findings in light of the child's pre-, peri-, and postnatal course is necessary in early neuropsychological assessment. Clinicians also must appreciate the necessity of obtaining á thorough physical examination (including hearing and vision screening) in conjunction with neurodevelopmental assessment. In general, medical/biological risk factors are associated with later perceptual-performance, neurological, gross motor, and perhaps quantitative abilities (particularly in premature infants). Subsequent high-prevalence/low-severity dysfunctions (learning disabilities, ADHDs, and behavior problems) have also been associated with medical/biological risk. These risk factors can also affect measures of cognitive function if the measure is a summary score, such as found with the McCarthy Scales General Cognitive Index (GCI) (Aylward, 1993; Aylward & Pfeiffer, 1991; Aylward, Verhulst, & Bell, 1989).

There are a variety of instruments that measure prenatal and perinatal medical risk (V. J. Molfese, 1989). Most reflect a combination of risk factors, as single factors in isolation probably are not significant, unless they are severe. These risk indices fall in one of two categories: the *complications approach* and the *optimality approach*. In the former, points are given cumulatively for the presence of risk factors. Complications scales use weighted values and have traditionally been employed to categorize children in terms of medical risk. However, it is difficult to determine weighting values. In the optimality approach (Prechtl, 1981), factors are identified that are most likely to predict positive outcomes. Optimality scales incorporate equal variable weights, the assumption being that because nonoptimal conditions rarely occur in isolation, a more serious condition will result in fewer optimal scores with this method. The rationale is that an optimal score (defined as the best possible score) on a particular medical risk item (e.g., absence of IVH or lack of mechanical ventilation) has a higher probability of later normal outcome than would the presence of a nonoptimal finding. The more optimal medical findings, the greater is the likelihood that medical factors would not have a detrimental effect on neuropsychological outcome. In infant and early childhood neuropsychology, the myriad of medical complications that would predispose an infant to being at biological risk should be summarized in some manner. Difficulties encountered when one considers medical variables include the following: pre- and perinatal complications are poorly defined, a distinction from normal is difficult to quantify, and the conditions may be present for various durations and in varying

Table 5.1. Sample of Medical Risk Indexes

Index	Author(s)	Description
Neonatal Medical Index	Korner et al. (1994)	Designed for preterm infants, particularly those < 1000 g versus > 1000 g. Graded I (best) to V (worst). Limited applicability for older gestational ages.
Obstetric Complications Scale (OCS)/Postnatal Complications Scale (PCS)	Littman & Parmelee (1978)	Based on Prechtl's optimality scoring; two scales but probably outdated because of medical advances. Conversion scores not clear.
Perinatal Risk Inventory (PERI)	Scheiner & Sexton (1991)	18 items, weighted 0–3 (best–worst). Scores totaled. Higher score = worse prognosis. Apgars, EEGs, gestational age, illness, etc.
Neurobiologic Risk Score (NBRS)	Brazy et al. (1991)	13 items; 0 = item absent, scores 1, 2, 4 (mild to severe). Apgars, ventilation, IVH, metabolic indicators. Not easily completed without thorough chart analysis. Focus on items that affect brain development.
Obstetric Optimality Scale	Touwen et al. (1980)	Based on Prechtl's model, contains 74 items, including measures of environment. Scored 1 or 0 and summed. Too lengthy in general.

degrees, from mild to severe. Some investigators suggest that the best gross measure of medical risk is *the number of days the child remains in the hospital after birth* (analogous to using maternal education as a measure of the environment). Some of the more common scales are listed in Table 5.1 (an excellent review of this topic is found in V. J. Molfese, 1989). The table is not exhaustive, as many scales (e.g., Hobel, Gyvarinen, & Okada, 1973) are dated and do not reflect current medical advances. Many authors have developed similar summary scores for individual studies (e.g., Aylward, 1993; Aylward et al., 1989).

EXAMPLES

■ A 2-year-old girl with significant expressive and receptive language delays comes from a high SES household. The *area* of function (language) is adequately evaluated at age 2, and the *environment* does not appear to be a negative influence. In this case, the child's *family and medical history*, including whether language problems have occurred in relatives, and assessment of hearing are critical. The prognosis for this child warrants concern. In contrast, had the same profile occurred in a child from a lower-SES, understimulating household, then *environmental effects* would assume more importance and be the prime focus of intervention. This would be the case because the area assessed (language) is typically influenced by the environment and the age (2 years) is when the effects become more pronounced.

■ Consider a 6-month-old (corrected age) infant, birth weight of 1000 g, who presents with increased tone of the lower extremities (including brisk patellar reflexes [knee jerk] and tight heel cords), and comes from a lower-SES household. In this case, *age* and *medical history* are particularly important, as many children born at this birth weight will demonstrate increased tone of the lower extremities over the first 6 months (*transient hypertonia*), which improves by 12 months of age. *Environment* is probably not important in this regard, because of the child's age and the *area of function* that is problematic (motor). Serial neurodevelopmental assessment would be necessary. However, the situation would be more worrisome if the child was 18 months old; because of the infant's age this would suggest an increased likelihood that the motor dysfunction would persist, again regardless of environmental circumstances.

In this overall evaluation procedure, the *risk route* model (Aylward & Kenny, 1979; see Chapter 2) would be applicable in that medical/biological, environmental/ psychosocial, and developmental/behavioral factors must be considered in combination. Moreover, biological, environmental, and established risks need to be considered as well.

"DEVELOPMENTAL BIAS"

One final general assessment consideration is that of developmental bias. Here, the ability to evaluate a given function or neuropsychological area is limited by three factors: (1) the "window" or time of assessment, (2) the developmental emergence of a specific function, and (3) the natural course of an "abnormal" finding (deviance). Concerning normal emergence, the clinician should consider the different areas of neuropsychological function as a series of progressively widening bands, starting thinly and gradually increasing in width with age. The rates of widening vary, depending on the specific neuropsychological function. Neurological function/intactness would be relatively wide very early on, as neurological functioning manifestations are obvious even in newborn evaluation. However, cognitive processes are not as pronounced during early infancy, but their manifestations progressively become more apparent (see Fig. 5.2). Therefore, in Fig. 5.2, the greater the width of the developmental band, the more prominent is the area of function and the greater is the likelihood that it can be assessed accurately. The situation is compounded further by developmental discontinuities in which the manifestations

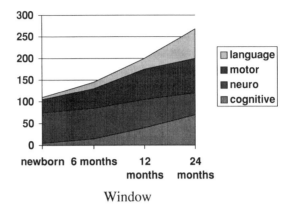

Window

Figure 5.2. Developmental bias ("normal" emergence).

(emergence and continuity) of a particular area (width of the band) may vary, depending on the time (window) it is assessed.

Similarly, in the case of abnormal indicators of deviance (Fig. 5.3), whether a deviant pattern is identified will depend on the progression and the window of testing. For example, hypertonicity may be evident early on but then undergo a "silent period." Hypotonicity, on the other hand, may not be evident until later, and then persist for quite some time. Ataxia would usually not be apparent until after the infant walks; tremors may be apparent very early on and then reemerge later. Thus, assessment is likened to shooting at a moving target; whether or not the shot is accurate depends on the size of the target, and when the shot is fired (see Figs. 5.2 and 5.3).

This issue probably is not as critical in neuropsychological assessment of older children because developmental change is not as rapid. The resultant developmental bands are more consistent with age, and deviations also are more stable.

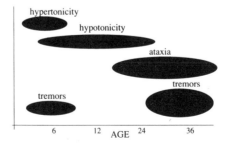

Figure 5.3. Developmental bias ("abnormal" deviance).

NEWBORN/NEONATAL ASSESSMENT

Over the last several decades, infant neuropsychological assessment has evolved from being neurologically based to more neurobehaviorally driven. This was particularly the case with newborn and neonatal neuropsychology. Reflexes, though still extremely important, were gradually augmented with more emphasis on movement and tone (neurological functions/intactness), expressive gross motor functions, and behavioral components (orientation to visual and auditory input, habituation to external stimuli, self-quieting activity, and level of consciousness [states]). Inclusion of more "neurobehavioral" items was necessary because the predictive utility of early neurological evaluations was modest at best. Evaluation of the infant's ability for self-organization, reactions to the environment, and other similar behaviors most likely taps into coordination of functional brain units, versus more circumscribed neurological channels. The purposes for early assessment also have varied and include: (1) estimation of gestational age (e.g., Ballard et al., 1991; Dubowitz, Dubowitz, & Goldberg, 1970), (2) maturity (Korner et al., 1994), (3) determination of current neurological intactness (Prechtl, 1977; Touwen, 1976), (4) prediction of later outcome (Aylward, Verhulst, & Colliver, 1985), (5) determination of the effects of exposure to drugs (Brazelton, 1973), and (6) determination of recovery from pre- or perinatal stress (Amiel-Tison, 1982).

The prime argument for implementation of newborn and neonatal neuropsychological assessment is that this is the only way to obtain an unrestricted view of the baby's functioning, before other factors obscure the underlying neurological and neurobehavioral intactness. MacKeith (1977) stated that although the infant's history tells us of risk, "only the neurological examination can tell the state of the brain's functioning." Moreover, he raised the question, "Why is it that, whilst for the first ten days of life we can detect dysfunction of the nervous system, once these early days of life are past, the windows through which we look into the nervous system often close and the brain functions normally and yet, after several months, dysfunction appears again?" (p. v).

Several considerations are particularly unique to newborn/neonatal assessment: 1) environmental conditions such as light and temperature, 2) body posture/positioning, 3) time since last feed, and 4) behavioral state. Newborns chill easily, and therefore examination on a heated bed often is required. Similarly, bright lighting interferes with accurate assessment of the baby's visual abilities. Both of these factors, although not to be disregarded in older babies, are much more critical early on. The infant's head also should be kept in midline to avoid asymmetric responses associated with primitive reflexes. Infants should be evaluated 2–3 hours after the last feed; the infant often is lethargic too soon after a feed, and irritable immediately before feeding.

Behavioral States

Behavioral states reflect the level of arousal in neonates, and the quality of elicited reflexes varies as a function of state. The delineation of states was originally accomplished by correlating observed behaviors in healthy, full-term newborns with measures of physiological function (Prechtl, 1968). States also have been evaluated in preterm infants (Aylward, 1981). Although there are subtle differences in the definition of states, they typically range from 1 (deep sleep) through 5 or 6 (crying). For example, Prechtl (1977) provided the following categorization:

- State 1: eyes closed, regular respiration, no movements
- State 2: eyes closed, irregular respiration, no gross movements (REM)
- State 3: eyes open, no gross movements
- State 4: eyes open, gross movements, no crying
- State 5: eyes open or closed, crying

Brazelton (1973) outlined the same two sleep states, but subdivided the "awake states" into three categories: drowsy or semidozing, alert with bright look, and eyes open, with a high activity level (fussy, but not crying). Regardless of the rating scheme, states generally progress from quiet sleep, active sleep, drowsiness, alert inactivity, waking activity, and crying. The significance of states resides in the fact that because the expression of neural mechanisms in the neonate is inconsistent, eliciting behaviors in specific states facilitates standardization. Optimum behavioral states for various neuropsychological items have been specified. For example, tone is decreased, but deep tendon reflexes are increased in state 2; in states 5 and 6, there is increased flexor tone of the upper extremities and increased extensor tone in the legs. States also enable assessment of mental activity; quiet, alert states are suggestive of CNS intactness, whereas continued irritability or lethargy may be indicative of CNS disruption.

Clinicians must also consider that repeated tests on several occasions during the neonatal period are much more valuable than a single assessment. This relates to the fact that repeated evaluations may depict a recovery curve, and also provide insight as to how recovery from the birth process or illness may affect the neonate's behavior. Because of the newborn's tendency to be easily fatigued, handling should be as efficient as possible. It is recommended that assessment be administered in "packages," depending on the infant's orientation: supine, upright, prone, and while being held. Actual areas of assessment include: (1) tone, (2) movements, (3) reaction type, (4) states, and (5) reflexes. Regardless of the area, keen *observation* is critical.

A brief listing of newborn/neonatal assessments is provided in Table 5.2. There is considerable overlap between instruments, and a good description of items common between the tests is contained in V. J. Molfese's review (1992)

Table 5.2. Neuropsychological Assessment Instruments for Neonates

Assessment	Authors	Ages
Infant Neurological Examination	Andre-Thomas et al. (1960)	0–12 months
Amiel-Tison's Neurologic Assessment	Amiel-Tison & Grenier (1986), Amiel-Tison et al. (1982)	0–12 months
Neonatal Neurodevelopment Examination	Allen & Capute (1989)	36–44 weeks (postmenstrual age)
Neurological Assessment of the Preterm and Fullterm Newborn Infant	Dubowitz & Dubowitz (1981)	Neonatal
Saint-Anne Dargassies' Neurological Examination	Saint-Anne Dargassies (1977)	Preterm and term
Brief Infant Neurobehavioral Optimality Scale	Aylward, Verhulst, & Colliver (1985)	Term
Prechtl Neurological Examination	Prechtl (1977), Prechtl & Beintema (1964)	Term
Parmelee Newborn Neurological Examination	Howard et al. (1976), Parmelee et al. (1974)	Term
Brazelton Neonatal Behavioral Assessment Scale	Brazelton (1973)	Term
Assessment of Preterm Infants' Behavior (APIB)	Als et al. (1982)	Preterm
Neurobehavioral Assessment of the Preterm Infant (NAPI)	Korner & Thom (1990)	Preterm
Revised Prechtl for Assessment of Preterm and Fullterm Infants	Aylward & Brown (1974)	Preterm–term
Graham Behavior Test for Neonates	Rosenblith (1974)	Newborn
Einstein Neonatal Neuro-Behavioral Assessment Scale (ENNAS)	Kurtzberg et al. (1979)	Newborn

and in Aylward (1988, pp. 240–241). A description of specific items frequently incorporated in newborn and neonatal assessment is found in Table 5.3. This listing is not exhaustive, but reflects means of assessing *proprioceptive, extero-ceptive,* and *nociceptive* neural networks. These neurobehavioral items are considered the most important and are contained in the most widely accepted neonatal neuropsychological examinations.

Neuropsychological function in this age range should be viewed as a series of major developmental landmarks. This series includes: maturation of individual processes, formulation of neural subsystems, coordination of these subsystems, adaptation of these coordinations to environmental demands (producing functional displays of behaviors), and development of higher cognitive processes. Simple, one-to-one relationships between underlying neural circuitry and observable behaviors appear to decrease with each progressive step. Correlations between these responses and medical/biological factors also decrease with maturation. Also, flexor tone increases, corresponding to an increase in gestational age; the younger the infant (prior to term), the more likely he or she will display extensor tone/posture. At birth, flexor tone predominates; as the infant develops more control, flexor tone becomes more balanced with extensor tone, this occurring in a cephalocaudal (head-to-toe) fashion.

A 15-item brief form, useful in clinical practice, was developed by Aylward, Verhulst, and Colliver (1985). Items included in this Brief Infant Neurobehavioral

Table 5.3. Neurological Item Groupings and Descriptions

Item	State	Description
Elicited		
Abdominal skin	2,3	Scratch with pin from side toward center of abdomen; all four quadrants. Response = quick contraction of abdominal musculature.
Palmar grasp	3,4	Place examiner's (E) finger into hands and gently press the palmar surface [never touch dorsal side]. Response = flexion of fingers around E's finger.
Plantar grasp	not 1,2	E presses thumbs against balls of infant's feet. Response = plantar flexion of all toes.
Babinski	any	Scratch sole of foot on lateral side, toes toward heel. Response = dorsal flexion of big toe, spreading of small toes.
Magnet response	3,4	Light pressure on soles; light contact with the feet while lower limbs extend. Response = extension of lower limbs.
Crossed extensor	3,4,5	Hold one leg and scratch sole repeatedly. Response = other leg flexes and then extends with adduction and fanning of toes.
Withdrawal	3	Gently scratch sole. Response = flexion of hip, knee, foot (often both legs).
Rooting/sucking	3,4,5	Stimulate corners of mouth with finger/put index finger in infant's mouth. Response = turn of head to stimulated side/sucking movements.
Trunk incurvation	3,4,5	Scratch slowly along paravertebral line, 3–4 cm from midline, from shoulder blades to buttocks. Response = trunk curves on stimulated side.
Placing	4	Baby held under the arms and around chest, dorsal part of foot touches tabletop. Response = foot is lifted and placed on the table.
Stepping	4,5	Hold upright, under arms and around chest. Soles of feet touch surface of table. Move forward to facilitate stepping. Response = stepping movements.
Stretch		
Arm/leg recoil	3,4	Both forearms are simultaneously extended at elbow and released/both legs are extended at knee and released. Response = brisk, symmetrical flexion of arms/legs.

Table 5.3. (*Continued*)

Item	State	Description
Scarf sign	3,4	Holding infant's wrist, arm gently moved across the chest toward opposite shoulder and ear. Response = elbow crosses body from either axillary line to not reaching midline on same side.
Tendon reflexes	3,4	Knee jerk—support lower limb, with index finger tap tendon below patella. Ankle jerk—press both thumbs with abrupt movement against distal part of soles of feet. Response = quick extension of knee, quick dorsiflexion of foot.
Arm/leg traction	3,4	Grasp infant's hands at wrists and pull slowly up to sitting position/grasp ankles and lift legs upwards and toward head. Response = arms/legs remain moderately flexed at elbow/knee throughout procedure. Angle in back of knee sometimes is referred to as the popliteal angle.
Resistance against passive movements	3,4	Range of movement and resistance are assessed in neck, trunk, shoulders, elbows, hips, knees, and ankles. Flexion and extension are measured. Response = moderate resistance and range are desirable.
Vertical tone	4,5	Infant held as in placing/stepping, with feet on surface. Response = lower limbs, trunk, head straighten.
Change in body axis		
Head control-sitting	4,5	Infant supported in sitting position. Response = head is held in upright position.
Pull-to-sit	4,5	Same as arm traction, emphasis on head control. Response = attempt to keep head in line with body.
Moro	3,4,5	Head held in hand and body supported by the lower arm of *E*. Other hand supports lower back and buttocks. Head is dropped a few centimeters with sudden movement. Response = infant abducts upper limbs and extends forearms and fingers; then adduction and flexion.
Rotation	3,4,5	Held in upright suspension. Spin baby slowly (90 degrees), supporting head if necessary. Response = head, eyes turn toward direction of turn.
Prone suspension	3,4,5	Suspend baby in prone suspension, hands around chest, infant's arms held freely. Response = infant shows antigravity posture.
Visual/auditory		
Orienting	3,4	Visual, auditory stimulation (voice, face, bull's-eye target, rattle) gently presented. Response = infant quiets, orients toward visual or auditory stimuli.
Acoustic/optic blink	2,3,4	Loud noise (bell) or bright light (penlight) suddenly presented. Response = infant blinks in response to auditory or visual stimulation. Frequent habituation after several presentations.
Non-elicited		

Spontaneous motor activity, tremors, crawling, head lifting when prone, side-to-side movements, posture, and crying are observed over the course of testing.

Optimality Scale are: knee-jerk, arm traction, head control in the pull-to-sit maneuver, resistance against passive movements (neck, trunk, shoulders, hips, knees), spontaneous motor activity (intensity, speed), headlifting prone, power of active movements, posture in prone suspension, placing, and stepping.

Abnormal Signs

In the optimality approach, the more "optimal" responses an infant displays, the better the prognosis is. Indicators of deviancy include hypertonia, hypotonia, brisk tendon reflexes, excessive axial (trunk) tone, clonus (repetitive responses to deep tendon items), tremors (low frequency/high amplitude), left/right discrepancies, excessive or few movements (hyper- or hypokinesis), predominant extensor tone, persistent asymmetric postures, frequent low-intensity responses, difficulty in arousing, consistent irritability (over several examinations), poor sucking (not related to feeding), and weak "vigor" in responses. Abnormal eye movements, and poor orientation to auditory or visual stimuli (e.g., visual tracking) also are important findings.

INFANT ASSESSMENT

During infancy (birth to 24 months; the neonatal period being the first 30 days after birth), functions defined as *neuropsychological* evolve from combined neurological and neurobehavioral functions to more discrete *developmental* and *neurological* categorizations. More specifically, there is gradual divergence of these two realms of functioning. Although development has an obvious neurological substrate, developmental functions are also influenced by environmental and experiential factors, and rely on the integration of behavioral units (versus the more one-to-one neurological reflex circuits). Therefore, it is helpful to view infant neuropsychological assessment in terms of neurological *and* developmental functions; grouping areas of strength and weakness into these categories aids in evaluation and prognosis, and perhaps even lends insight into the etiology of problems. As previously indicated, more neurologically based functions are influenced by medical/biological factors, whereas other functions such as verbal expressive or cognitive processes are subject to a more complex array of influences. Neurological functions are more localized, and developmental acquisitions migrate toward the "behavioral" side of "brain–behavior" relationships (V. J. Molfese, 1991). Moreover, one should consider neurological abnormality in terms of its *functional significance*. For example, decreased tone of the lower extremities at 9 months of age is nonoptimal neurologically, but might not have a significant developmental impact if the child is adequately able to get to a sitting position, crawl, and pull up on furniture. Similarly, tight heel cords (decreased ankle dorsiflexion) again are nonoptimal, but assume less importance if the child is able to place his or her foot flatly on the table surface and demonstrate adequate acquisition of motor milestones such as walking with support or independently.

There are very few tests *specifically* designed to evaluate neuropsychological functions in infancy. Most tests are developmentally oriented, but extrapolations regarding neuropsychological function can be made. This approach was first outlined by Aylward (1988), and an updated summary is found in Table 5.4. At this age, assessments cluster in the *receptive, expressive,* and *cognitive processes* groupings. Sensorimotor skills are generally emphasized; these include visual motor/integrative, fine motor-constructive, and gross motor functions. Visual-perceptual abilities are also heavily weighted. However, assessment of neurological functions/intactness has been an underemphasized area. In fact, only the Milani-Comparetti Neurodevelopmental Screening Examination (Milani-Comparetti & Gidoni, 1967a, b) originally involved assessment of neurodevelopmental function. This prompted Aylward (1988) to underscore the need for early neuropsychological instruments and forward the Early Neuropsychologic Optimality Rating Scales (ENORS; Aylward, 1994; Aylward et al., 1994) as a possible solution. The ENORS served as the early prototype for the Bayley Infant Neurodevelopmental Screener (BINS; Aylward, 1995).

Table 5.4. Infant Evaluation Instruments with Neuropsychological Applications

Test	Neuropsychological/ neurodevelopmental	Developmental	Author
Gesell Developmental Schedules	N	Y	Knobloch & Pasamanick (1974), Knobloch et al. (1980)
Bayley Scales of Infant Development/Bayley Scales of Infant Development II	N	Y	Bayley (1969), Bayley (1993)
Griffiths Mental Developmental Scale	N	Y	Griffiths (1970)
Milani-Comparetti Neurodevelopmental Screening Examination	Y	N	Milani-Comparetti & Gidoni (1967)
Early Neuropsychologic Optimality Rating Scales (ENORS)	Y	N	Aylward et al. (1988a, b, 1994)
Bayley Infant Neurodevelopmental Screener (BINS)	Y	N	Aylward (1995)
Infant Mullen Scales of Early Learning (Infant MSEL)	N	Y	Mullen (1989)

ENORS

Six versions of the ENORS have been developed (Aylward, 1994; Aylward et al., 1994), applicable to the key ages of 3, 6, 9, 12, 18, and 24 months (*conceptional age*, ± 1 month). Each ENORS version contains from 16 to 22 component items, grouped under the headings outlined in Table 5.5. A summary of functions evaluated by the six ENORS versions is found in Table 5.6. Clinicians and researchers who administer the ENORS must be well versed in "normal" development, as this is the basis from which deviations in neuropsychological function can

Table 5.5. Sample ENORS Items

Version(s)	Item	Optimal	Nonoptimal
I. Basic neurological function/intactness			
3	Primitive reflexes present (asymmetric tonic neck response, palmar grasp, plantar grasp)	Yes	No
6	Presence of normal protective reactions (downwards parachute reaction)	Yes	No
9	Presence of normal protective reactions (forwards, downwards, sideways parachute)	Yes	No
12	Hypotonia/hypertonia (trunk, extremities, brisk deep tendon reflexes)	No	Yes
18/24	No excessive drooling or motor overflow (mirroring)	Yes	No
II. Receptive functions			
3/6	Appropriate responses to auditory stimuli (orients, turns head)	Yes	No
9	Follows simple commands/gestures	Yes	No
12	Follows simple commands/gestures and understands words	Yes	No
18	Follows directions	Yes	No
24	Points to four pictures named by examiner/points to six body parts	Yes	No
IIIa. Expressive functions—fine motor			
3	Makes arm movements toward objects, may reach and make contact	Yes	No
6	Rakes small objects (pellet)	Yes	No
9	Inferior pincer grasp	Yes	No
12	Neat pincer grasp	Yes	No
18	Can imitate crayon strokes	Yes	No
24	Stacks four cubes, imitates crayon strokes	Yes	No
IIIb. Expressive functions—oral motor			
3	Makes sounds (vowels, cooing)	Yes	No
6	Babbles/appropriate sounds for age (vowels, consonants)	Yes	No
9/12	Says mama/dada, babbles	Yes	No
18	Uses words with meaning	Yes	No
24	Speech is 50% intelligible	Yes	No

Table 5.5. (*Continued*)

Version(s)	Item	Optimal	Nonoptimal
IIIc. Expressive functions—gross motor			
3	Elevates self in prone position/head at 45 degree angle	Yes	No
6	Sits with propping/rolls over	Yes	No
9	Crawls/creeps/sits	Yes	No
12	Age-appropriate gait/ambulation	Yes	No
18	Ascent/descent stairs holding on	Yes	No
24	Jumps (both feet off floor)	Yes	No
IV. Processing			
3	Regards objects in hands	Yes	No
6	Looks for fallen objects	Yes	No
9	Simple imitative abilities (suspends ring, scribbling)	Yes	No
12	Simple problem solving skills	Yes	No
18	Good appreciation of object permanency (finds hidden object under cup)	Yes	No
24	Completes form board	Yes	No
V. Mental activity			
3	Goal-directed behavior (plays with rattle, objects to mouth)	Yes	No
6/9	Attentive to procedures	Yes	No
12	Goal-directed behavior (persistence, puts three cubes in cup)	Yes	No
18	Average activity level for age	Yes	No
24	Goal-directed behavior (persists in attempt to obtain object, perform an activity with toy)	Yes	No

Source: From Aylward, G. P. (1994). Update on early developmental neuropsychologic assessment: The Early Neuropsychologic Optimality Rating Scales. In M. G. Tramontana & S. R. Hooper (Eds.), *Advances in child neuropsychology* (Vol. 2, pp. 172–200). Springer-Verlag. Used with permission.

be compared. Items are scored by three methods: observation, elicitation, and caregiver report. The proportion of items scored by each method varies by age. The infant is placed supine, prone, held upright, is seated on the caretaker's lap, or ambulates, again depending on age. For example, at 3 months most items are

Table 5.6. Summary of Functions Evaluated by the Six ENORS Versions

	3	6	9	12	18	24
I. Basic neurological function/intactness[a]						
1. Primitive reflexes[b]	X	X	X	X		
2. Asymmetries	X	X	X	X		
3. Head control	X	X	X	X	X	
4. Muscle tone	X	X	X	X		
5. Abnormal indicators	X	X	X	X		
6. Protective reactions		X	X	X		
7. Drooling/motor overflow					X	X

Table 5.6. (*Continued*)

	3	6	9	12	18	24
II. Receptive functions						
1. Auditory	X	X	X	X		
2. Visual	X	X	X	X	X	X
3. Visual tracking		X	X			
4. Verbal receptive			X	X	X	X
5. Understands body parts					X	X
III. Expressive functions						
A. Fine motor/oral motor						
1. Reaching behavior	X	X				
2. Hands open/midline behaviors	X	X	X	X	X	
3. Prehension skills		X	X	X	X	
4. Eye–hand coordination			X	X	X	X
5. Fine motor control					X	X
6. Vocalizations/verbalizations	X	X	X	X	X	X
7. Names objects/pictures						X
B. Gross motor						
1. Elevates self-prone	X					
2. Supports weight	X					
3. Coordinated movement	X	X	X	X		
4. Sitting/rolls over		X	X			
5. Crawling/preambulation			X			
6. Ambulation				X	X	X
7. Throwing/kicking					X	X
8. Ascends stairs					X	X
9. Jumps						X
IV. Processing						
1. Social smile	X					
2. Regards objects	X					
3. Object permanence		X	X	X	X	X
4. Imitative abilities		X	X	X	X	
5. Problem solving		X	X	X	X	X
6. Form boards						X
V. Mental activity						
1. Goal-directed behaviors	X	X	X	X	X	X
2. Attentiveness	X	X	X	X	X	X
3. Activity level	X	X	X	X	X	X
4. Persistent crying/irritability	X					

[a]Item cluster.
[b]Component item.
Source: From Aylward, G. P. (1994). Update on early developmental neuropsychologic assessment: The Early Neuropsychologic Optimality Rating Scales. In M. G. Tramontana & S. R. Hooper (Eds.), *Advances in child neuropsychology* (Vol. 2, pp. 172–200). Springer-Verlag. Used with permission.

observational; by 24 months, the number is reduced to less than one-third, the vast majority being elicited by the examiner. Similarly, with increasing age, more items are administered while the infant is seated on the caretaker's lap. Also, although component items may be evaluated at several ages, the individual parts and/or scoring criteria may differ. For example, with the primitive reflexes component item at 3 months, item parts such as asymmetric neck posturing, and palmar and plantar grasps should be *present*; however, at 6 months these should be *absent*.

ENORS Item Groupings

- The ENORS-3 is the newest version. It was developed to complete the infancy assessment package, with the realization that predictive validity may be low because of issues such as recovery of function, the possibility that medical complications may still exert a strong effect at this age, and the transitory nature of certain early neurological abnormalities. The ENORS-3 contains 20 items, with the Basic Neurological Function/Intactness category having the most components (5) followed by Mental Activity (4). In regard to assessment with the ENORS-3, it should be noted that decreased tone often improves between 3 and 6 months, perhaps because energy expended in recovery from a medical condition weakens the child, and takes its toll on this particular area of function. Medical variables are also likely to influence gross motor expressive items, primarily because of the "vigor" required for their expression. Goal-directed behaviors and attentiveness may be the most prognostically useful items contained in this instrument.
- The ENORS-6 contains 21 component items, with Basic Neurological Function/Intactness and Fine Motor/Oral Motor Expressive clusters receiving the most emphasis (each with 6 item parts). Processing items become more important and are prognostically more significant, because they incorporate integration of several functional units (e.g., imitation, object permanence). It is not unusual at this age to find an increase in tone in the lower extremities in children born at young gestational ages. Although such findings are nonoptimal, their significance is lessened if the hypertonicity is restricted (i.e., is not found in the axial musculature) and movement is coordinated. On the ENORS-6, a cutoff value of 75 or 80% optimal responses (computed as: number optimal/[number optimal + number nonoptimal]) appears to be most useful in terms of sensitivity and specificity (see Aylward, 1994).
- The ENORS-9 (the first of the ENORS versions) contained 24 items (Aylward et al., 1988a) , but item total was reduced to 22 (the Bayley MDI and PDI were deleted). Item groupings are listed in Table 5.6. Of

interest, however, is the finding that the component items Basic Neurological Function/Intactness, Expressive Functions, and Mental Activity are particularly predictive of the McCarthy Scales General Cognitive Index at 36 months; Fine and Gross Motor Expressive, Processing, and Mental Activity item clusters are associated with 36-month motor function. A cutoff score of 85% optimal is most useful in regard to cognitive and motor function; 75% optimal is most predictive of neurological function.

■ The ENORS-12 contains 22 component items, with Basic Neurological Function/Intactness and Fine Motor/Oral Motor Expressive item clusters having the largest representation (6 and 5 items, respectively). Processing and Mental Activity clusters also receive increased emphasis. A 75% cutoff value is recommended for this version.

■ The ENORS-18 (the second version to be developed; Aylward et al., 1988b) contains a significant loading of Fine Motor/Oral Motor, Processing, and Mental Activity items (Table 5.6). In line with the schedule of developmental acquisitions, the ENORS-18 has increased emphasis on verbal and processing functions. A cutoff value of 80% optimal has been cited as providing the best sensitivity and specificity values in regard to later cognitive outcome, however, 70 and 75% cutoff values are also acceptable (Aylward et al., 1988b).

■ The ENORS-24 contains 16 composite items (each with 1- to 4-item parts). More emphasis is placed on language function (receptive and expressive) than in earlier versions of the ENORS. A 65% cutoff yields the best sensitivity and specificity.

In summary, Basic Neurological Function/Intactness items are important primarily during the first year, visual receptive items are important throughout infancy, and verbal receptive skills increase in significance from 9 months onward. Mental Activity items are emphasized consistently throughout infancy. Although different functions assume differential importance over the six key ENORS ages, each area is evaluated to some degree, thereby enhancing conceptual continuity.

The ENORS-6, -12, and -24 recently have been shown to be highly predictive of later outcome at 36 months of age (Aylward et al., 1994). Using hierarchical regression, the ENORS versions accounted for 43–68% of the variance on the McCarthy Scales of Children's Abilities subscales. In children having an optimal ENORS and SES-Composite Index (a six-item measure of the environment; Aylward, Dunteman, Hatcher, Gustafson, & Widmayer, 1985), 83–97% were later "normal," depending on age and area of function. Using odds ratios, an optimal ENORS-6 increased the likelihood of normal 3-year outcome by 2.4 to 10.7 times; odds ratios ranging from 9.85 to 90.1 and from 10.5 to 54.5 were found for optimal ENORS-12 and ENORS-24 scores, respectively. Moreover, if both the ENORS and environmental measures are optimal, then the likelihood of normal 36-month outcome is quite high.

BINS

The BINS (Aylward, 1995) is the outgrowth of the ENORS, and enables assessment of posture, tone, movement, developmental status and basic neurological intactness in infants from 3 to 24 months. There are six item sets: 3–4, 5–6, 7–10, 11–15, 16–20, and 21–24 months, each containing 11–13 items. Four conceptual areas are assessed (see Chapter 1): Basic Neurological Function/Intactness, Receptive Functions, Expressive Functions, and Cognitive Processes (combined Cognitive Processes and Mental Activity from the ENORS). The conceptual clusters are not thought to be orthogonal; it is expected that for any one item, the abilities represented in any one cluster are involved along with abilities from another cluster. The BINS takes 10 minutes to administer. Caregiver report is allowed on only certain items, and only one caregiver report is allowed for any conceptual grouping (a total of two for any BINS administration). The BINS is based on the optimality concept, the main premise being that prediction of later positive outcomes by early optimal findings is more accurate than is prediction of later negative outcomes by early nonoptimal findings. The optimality approach yields three classification groupings: *low risk*, *moderate risk*, and *high risk*. The classifications groupings are used to determine the likelihood of later developmental problems. Items are scored *optimal* (1) or *nonoptimal* (0) and are summed to provide a total score. By using different cutoff scores, flexibility is afforded examiners in terms of deciding which infants need further assessment. Comparing a child's performance on items in the four conceptual clusters provides the opportunity to determine whether the problems are global versus specific, and to define areas of function that require more detailed evaluation. The BINS also assists the examiner in making initial determinations as to whether the dysfunction is more restricted to neurological findings (e.g., increased tone), developmental milestones (walking, fine motor), or both areas.

The BINS is not a "mini-Bayley II"; it emphasizes a process approach by considering how an ability is expressed, rather than simply whether the ability is exhibited. The BINS correlates moderately well with the BSID-II, and in fact the correlations are comparable to the associations between the original BSID and the BSID-II.

In a recent longitudinal study, correlations between the 6-, 12-, and 24-month BINS scores were moderate, indicating that there was approximately a 50% overlap in variance. This finding suggests that the different BINS versions share continuity as well as unique aspects. Moreover, there was a statistically significant difference between the 36-month McCarthy Scales GCI, and the Verbal, Perceptual-Performance, and Motor Scale scores of children falling into the low-, moderate-, and high-risk BINS groupings at 6, 12, and 24 months of age. Risk status classifications were fairly consistent over time as well; if change did occur, it typically was the result of children shifting from moderate to high risk, or moderate to low risk. High- and low-risk status classifications were quite stable (Aylward, Verhulst, & Bell, 1996). More recent data (Aylward, unpublished)—in which the moderate-risk category was separated and combined with either the high-risk (moderate/high) or low-risk grouping (moderate/low) odds ratios predicting later, "normal" development—ranged from 2.5 to 10.5.

Milani-Comparetti Neurodevelopmental Screening Examination

Although neuropsychological information can be readily gleaned from developmental tests (Table 5.4), true infant neuropsychological assessment should also include neurological items. The Milani-Comparetti examination (Milani-Comparetti & Gidoni, 1967) offers such an opportunity; it is a "motoscopic" assessment (from the Italian *motoscopia*, meaning "observation of movement"). It requires 5–10 minutes to administer, and can be incorporated into developmental assessment of infants from birth to 24 months in a complementary fashion. This particular instrument is emphasized here because of its utility and easy adaptability. Items are grouped into two categories: (1) *spontaneous behavior* (postural control of the head and body, active movement) and (2) *evoked responses* (primitive reflexes, righting reactions, parachute reactions, and tilting reactions). Although discussion of the entire examination is beyond the scope of this section, selected items are briefly addressed below in order to underscore some general, neuropsychological principles and progressions.

Spontaneous Behavior

Postural Control—Head. When held vertically, head control increases over the first month, with full control being evident by the 4th month (*body held vertical* item). When prone, the 2-month-old keeps her head in line with her body when lifting; at 4 months the head should be held 45 degrees from the table surface, and at 6 months, the angle should be 90 degrees (*body lying prone* item). In the *body lying supine* item, the infant should lift her head (flexion) by 5 months (in a "sit-up"-like maneuver). In the *body pulled from supine* item, the head is kept in line with the trunk from 4 to 5 months, and at ≥ 5 months, the infant will lead her body with her head.

Postural Control—Body. In terms of *sitting*, at 6 months, the infant can sit while propping; prior to that (4 months), the infant can straighten the back down to the L3 (lumbar) level. At 7 months the baby can sit without support, albeit in an unsteady fashion. Trunk control develops in a cephalocaudal progression. In prone, at 3½ months the infant rests on his elbows, at 4 months on his hands, and at 7–9 months, his hands and knees (quadriped). By 10 months, the child supports his weight in a plantigrade manner (hands and feet in a "bearwalking" fashion). Standing evolves in a manner that underscores a significant principle in infant neuropsychology, namely, that certain behaviors may be present early on in development, but then disappear, only to emerge again later, but under control of a different area of the brain (subcortical to cortical). The infant can support his weight for the first 1–2 months, but then his legs might collapse when his feet contact the table surface (*astasia*). This may persist up to 5 months, at which time support reemerges. At first the child will stand with trunk forward and hips flexed, but by 10 months, he should stand erect. A similar profile is found with locomotion: reflexive, automatic stepping occurs over the first 1–1½ months, and then ceases; it reemerges again during precursory walking. Ambulation also is accompanied by a *high*, then *medium*, and, finally, *low guard* (referring to arms held up or out to the sides for balance).

Evoked Responses

Primitive Reflexes. Another major infant neuropsychological principle is found in the consideration of primitive reflexes. These should be present early on (being mediated by lower brain centers), but with increasing cortical maturation, these should be suppressed and integrated with postural reactions. Continuation of primitive reflexes beyond the time that they "normally" would subside is considered indicative of CNS dysfunction. On the Milani-Comparetti, the hand grasp should disappear by 3–3½ months, asymmetric tonic neck posturing by 4 months, Moro by 4 months, and foot grasp by 9 months.

Righting Reactions. The *head in space* item is particularly useful. When the infant is held vertically, she is tilted to each side, as well as forwards and backwards. Adjustment of the head so that it remains upright should occur, beginning at approximately 1½ months of age. Similarly, when held in the sagittal plane (*prone suspension*) the baby will straighten her body "like an arrow" from 2 or 3 months onwards.

Parachute Reactions. The child is held under the arms in a vertical suspension and then is lowered rapidly to imitate a falling sensation. By 4 months, the normal child will straighten his legs and spread his feet outward (*downwards parachute reaction*). In the *sideways parachute*, the child is sitting and then pushed so that he loses balance; by 6 months, the normal infant will try to protect himself from falling by extending his arm and hand on the body side moving toward the surface.

In the *forwards parachute* reaction, the infant is held under the arms at midthorax and then is tilted forward suddenly toward the table surface. By 7 months the arms are straightened and fingers extended. Finally, with the *backwards parachute* reaction, the infant's ability to protect himself from falling backwards is tested in much the same way as the sideways parachute. Children 9 months and older will react by extending both hands outward or rotating to either side.

Therefore, items from the Milani-Comparetti can be added to developmental tests so as to provide a broader neuropsychological asssessment, and in fact, many are included in the ENORS.

In summary, only a few evaluation instruments are specifically designed to assess neuropsychological function in infancy. However, neuropsychological information can be gleaned from other developmentally oriented instruments. Combination of developmental and neurological data is routinely necessary when tests developed for other purposes are employed in neuropsychological assessment.

EARLY CHILDHOOD ASSESSMENT

Most traditional child neuropsychological batteries such as the Halstead Neuropsychological Test Battery for Children (ages 9–14 years), the Reitan–Indiana Battery (5–9 years), or the Luria–Nebraska Neuropsychological Battery for Children (8–12 years) are simply not applicable for preschoolers (3–5 years). Excessive length and limitations inherent in scaling tasks downward from adults preclude a "neuropsychological battery" approach. Even though additional subtests for younger children have been included in an effort to broaden applicability, neuropsychological tests in this range are more closely aligned to developmental, versus adult neuropsychological models, in a "bottom-up" rather than "top-down" approach. It cannot be assumed that tests that have validated brain–behavior relationships in adults with known lesions will show similar results with children. Therefore, clinicians should not make the assumption that a scaled-down version of an adult or even later-childhood test may necessarily be a measure of the same brain–behavior patterns as in adults.

Moreover, less emphasis is placed on localization because subtle CNS dysfunction is more difficult to determine, and functional systems of young children are less rigidly circumscribed and more capable of reorganization. Also, the preschool child who has CNS dysfunction simply has never experienced "normal" brain functioning. Therefore, the "chain" of dysfunction and subsequent neural integration may differ markedly; disruptions in function at different levels of the "chain" may produce similar behavioral phenotypes initially, but these can evolve into markedly different presentations with increasing age.

Again drawing on Luria's (1973) theory of brain development, at age 2 years, there is functional maturation of the secondary cortical areas (responsible for processing incoming information) and progressive lateralization of function occurs. The secondary cortical areas allow for synthesizing and acting on information received from subcortical and primary cortical areas. Therefore, over the first 5 years, the secondary cortical areas are the primary sites of learning. The tertiary cortical areas (overlapping zones that integrate information from secondary areas) and the prefrontal areas gradually develop from ages 4 to 7 years, and, with increasing age, play a greater role in learning and behavior. Therefore, the underlying cortical substrate that governs learning and behavior changes over infancy and early childhood, further mitigating against the use of adult models (which are often based on tertiary functions) in this age range.

Available test instruments that are applicable to early childhood neuropsychological assessment can be grouped into two areas: *intelligence/developmental tests* and *neurodevelopmental evaluation instruments*. Available tests are listed in Table 5.7. Again, this listing is not exhaustive.

Intelligence and developmental tests contain tasks that have neuropsychological applications; unfortunately, the former typically do not contain neuromotor components that are necessary to provide complete neuropsychological assessment. Therefore, clinicians may need to select tests from multiple evaluation instruments, to ensure that all neuropsychological functions are sampled adequately. Again, often it is the interpretive conceptual framework that makes the assessment "neuropsychological."

Clinicians who employ intelligence tests in early childhood neuropsychological assessment should be aware that many preschool IQ tests have weak test floors. As a result, it is difficult to distinguish between average, low average,

Table 5.7. Early Childhood Test Instruments with Neuropsychological Applications

Test	Ages	Authors
NEPSY	3–12 yr	Korkman et al. (1997)
Miller Assessment for Preschoolers (MAP)	2.9–6 yr	Miller (1988)
FirstSTEP: Screening Test for Evaluating Preschoolers	2.9–6 yr	Miller (1993)
Kaufman Assessment Battery for Children (K-ABC)	2½–12 yr	Kaufman & Kaufman (1983)
Bayley Scales of Infant Development-II	1–42 mo	Bayley (1993)
Differential Ability Scales	2½–18 yr	Elliott (1990)
McCarthy Scales of Childrens Abilities (MSCA)	2½–8½ yr	McCarthy (1972)
Mullen Scales of Early Learning (MSEL)	2–5½ yr	Mullen (1984)
Wechsler Preschool and Primary Scale of Intelligence (WPPSI-R)	3–7¼ yr	Wechlser (1989)
Stanford-Binet Fourth Edition (SB-4)	2–adult	Thorndike et al. (1986)
Leiter International Performance Scale-R	2–21 yr	Roid & Miller (1997)

and borderline performance. Degrees of mental retardation also cannot be easily differentiated. Further complicating the situation, summary scores generally increase by three to five points per decade, thereby affecting norms on older tests (e.g., Flanagan & Alfonso, 1995).

In early childhood or preschool neuropsychological assessment, clinicians must ensure that a broad range of functions is measured, and that this measurement is accurate. Recommended functions or neuropsychological systems to be included in early childhood assessment are found in Table 5.8. Use of this framework allows flexibility and enables the clinician to select complete instruments, particular subtests, or combinations of subtests, depending on the purpose of the evaluation. The framework can be applied to "complete" (self-contained) neuropsychological instruments or to other developmental or intelligence tests.

Table 5.8. Functions to Be Assessed in Early Childhood Neuropsychology

---

I. Basic neurological functions-intactness/neural foundations
    - reflexes
    - motor inhibition
    - awareness of sensations (position, movement, touch)
    - asymmetries
    - observation of abnormal indicators (postures, movements, signs)
    - balance (vestibular function)

II. Receptive functions
    A. Visual
        - visual perception (matching)
        - spatial relations
        - visual discrimination
    B. Auditory/language/verbal
        - auditory discrimination
        - language processing
        - comprehension
    C. Tactile
        - finger writing
        - tactile discrimination of objects

III. Expressive functions
    A. Oral motor/verbal
        - articulation
        - rhythmic oral motor sequencing
        - fluency
        - tongue movements
        - rhyming
        - verbal analogies
        - sentence, word, number repetition

Table 5.8. (*Continued*)

   B. Fine motor/sensorimotor/visuo-motor
- fine motor speed
- fine motor dexterity
- graphomotor skills
- left/right discrimination (laterality)
- sequential hand movements/alternating movements

   C. Gross motor
- body in space
- coordination (arms, legs)
- gross motor imitation (postures, movements)

IV. Cognitive processes/cognition/executive functions/learning

   A. Memory
- auditory temporal-sequential organization (words, sentences, lists, digits)
- visual memory (faces, objects, positions of objects)
- visual sequencing
- word retrieval
- passage/story memory
- cross-modal memory
- short term/long term

   B. Thinking/reasoning/learning
- problem solving/logical reasoning
- verbal abstracting (analogies)
- nonverbal abstracting (matrices)
- seriation/classification
- number concepts
- judgment
- planning
- associative learning

   C. Mental activity
- attention (selective, sustained)
- vigilance
- conceptual tracking/concentration
- inhibition (impulse control)
- alertness
- cognitive flexibility

Self-Contained Neuropsychological Assessment Instruments

■ The new NEPSY (Korkman, Kirk, & Kemp,1997) is a comprehensive neuropsychological instrument applicable for children ages 3–12. The NEPSY is based on a neuropsychological model and enables identification of deficiencies that interfere with a child's learning. Five functional domains are assessed: (1) *executive functions* (attention, planning, problem solving, vigilance, inhibition), (2) *language and communica-*

tion (word recognition, repetition of nonsense words, demand naming, production of oral motor sequences), (3) *sensorimotor functions* (tactile input, fine motor speed, imitation of hand positions, sequential movements, pencil skills), (4) *visuospatial functions* (judgment of position and directionality, copying two-dimensional geometric figures, reconstruction of three-dimensional designs), and (5) *learning and memory* (memory for words, pictures, faces, lists [immediate and delayed], narrative memory [free and cued recall]). The full NEPSY, a core set of items, or selected subtests can be administered. Time requirements appear appropriate for preschool-age children, ranging from 1 hour for the complete NEPSY, 30 minutes for the core tests, to approximately 10 minutes for individual subtests. The NEPSY includes items from virtually all of the functional areas included in Table 5.8.

■ The Miller Assessment for Preschoolers (MAP; Miller, 1988) is designed to identify preschoolers who are at risk for developmental delay, being applicable from ages 2.9 to 6 years. However, the test instrument has definite neuropsychological underpinnings. Items are grouped into five performance areas: (1) Neural Foundations, (2) Coordination, (3) Verbal, (4) Nonverbal, and (5) Complex Tasks. Assessed abilities fall into three main conceptual categories:

☐ *Sensory and motor.* This includes Neural Foundations and Coordination. The former consists of basic motor tasks and awareness of sensations (position, movement, touch). Many of these items are included in the standard neurological examination (stereogenesis, finger localization, hand-nose, Romberg). The Coordination subtests measure gross, fine, and oral motor functions (tower building, tongue movements, articulation, walking on a line, rapid alternating movements).

☐ *Cognitive.* Included in this category are Verbal and Nonverbal areas. The verbal items evaluate memory, sequencing, comprehension, association, and verbal expression (general information, following directions, sentence and digit repetition). Nonverbal functions assessed include memory, sequencing, and visual performance (block tapping, object memory, puzzles).

☐ *Combined abilities.* This area combines sensory, motor, and cognitive abilities that are required for interpretation of spatial-visual information (block designs, mazes, draw-a-person, imitation of postures).

The MAP has three color-coded diagnostic areas: *red* (< 5th percentile for the child's age group), *yellow* (between the 6th and 25th percentiles), and *green*

(> 25th percentile). This test is useful in identifying mild and moderate "preacademic" problems that have a neuropsychological basis, and fits nicely with the framework outlined in Table 5.8.

- The FirstSTEP (Miller, 1993) is a 15-minutes screener for the MAP. Twelve subtests are arranged in the five domains listed above for the MAP. A *composite score* consists of information obtained in three areas: Cognition, Communication, and Motor. Children are classified as falling within normal limits, questionable (mild to moderate delays), or at risk (significant delays). Although the age range is 2.9–6 years, some anecdotal evidence suggests that the floor may be too difficult for 3-year-olds with mild to moderate neurodevelopmental problems.

- The Kaufman Assessment Battery for Children (K-ABC, Kaufman & Kaufman, 1983) is a battery of tests designed to measure intelligence and achievement in children from 2½ to 12½ years. However, the test distinguishes *sequential* and *simultaneous* processing based on neuropsychological theory; emphasis is placed on the *process* used to solve a problem (either linear/analytic/sequential or gestalt/holistic/simultaneous) rather than the *content* of the task. Each task on the Sequential Processing Scale is solved by arranging the input in a sequential or serial order (hand movements, number recall, word order); this process is closely related to school-oriented skills such as memorization of number facts, lists of spelling words, phonics, or understanding sequences of events. The Simultaneous Processing Scale involves spatial, analogic, and organizational tasks. Input is integrated and synthesized simultaneously to produce a solution (identification of an object based on seeing only a part, face recognition, gestalt closure, two-dimensional shape assembly, and spatial memory). This process is related to school tasks such as learning shapes of letters and numbers, deriving meaning from pictures such as maps, and acquiring a "sight" vocabulary. A group of tests can be combined to produce a "nonverbal" score (face recognition, hand movements, triangles, spatial memory).

The K-ABC produces two meaningful factors before the age of 4 years: simultaneous and sequential. At this age the Expressive Vocabulary, Faces and Places, and Riddles are best interpreted as measures of simultaneous processing; Arithmetic is primarily a sequential subtest (see Aylward, 1994). This test is particularly useful in testing children with hearing or language impairment. It does not adequately measure the Basic Neurological Functions-Intactness/Neural Foundations area; all other areas are involved to some degree.

Other Tests Containing Neuropsychological Tasks

■ The Bayley Scales of Infant Development-II (BSID-II; Bayley, 1993) is applicable through 42 months of age and therefore is also included in the early childhood section. As with infant assessment, the BSID-II test results also can be interpreted within a neuropsychological framework. Use of item sets from the Mental and Motor scales enables assessment of all four functional areas outlined in Table 5.7, particularly if incidental observation is employed.

■ The Differential Ability Scales (DAS; Elliott, 1990) are applicable from 2½ to 17 years, 11 months, but are particularly useful in the late toddler and early childhood range. On the DAS, a *composite score* based on reasoning and conceptual abilities is derived, namely, the General Conceptual Ability Score (GCA). In addition, Verbal Ability and Nonverbal Ability Cluster Scores are produced; this allows for three levels of interpretation: the GCA, cluster scores, and subtest scores. From ages 2–6 to 3–5 there are four core tests (block building, picture similarities, naming vocabulary, verbal comprehension) and two diagnostic tests (recall of digits, recognition of pictures). From ages 3–6 to 5–11, there are six core tests (copying, pattern construction, early number concepts are added) and five diagnostic tests (block building, matching letterlike forms, recall of digits, recall of objects, recognition of pictures). Although the DAS allows for neuropsychological interpretation, Basic Neurological Functions (I), Gross Motor Expressive (III-C), and Mental Activity (IV-C) areas are not assessed adequately with sole use of this instrument.

■ The McCarthy Scales of Children's Abilities (MSCA, McCarthy, 1972) essentially bridges developmental and IQ tests (Aylward, 1994), and is most useful in the 3- to 5-year age range (the age range is 2½–8½ years). A total of 18 tests is involved, divided into five categories: *verbal* (five tests), *perceptual-performance* (seven tests), *quantitative* (three tests), *motor* (five tests), and *memory* (four tests). Several tests are found on two scales. The verbal, perceptual-performance, and quantitative scales are combined to yield a General Cognitive Index (GCI). A feature that makes the MSCA attractive to the clinician is the ability to produce a profile of functioning (with age equivalents). Although the MSCA does not adequately measure Basic Neurological Functions (I), it does have a useful Gross Motor component. On the negative side, the test is 25 years old, and the norms are somewhat dated.

■ The Mullen Scales of Early Learning (MSEL; Mullen, 1984) assesses the 2- to 5½-year-old's learning abilities and patterns in multiple developmental domains. Neuropsychologically, the MSEL measures unevenness in the child's learning, with particular emphasis on differentiation of visual and auditory learning. Moreover, the MSEL provides information that enables the clinician to differentiate receptive or expressive problems in either the visual or auditory domain by use of four scales: Visual Receptive Organization (VRO), Visual Expressive Organization (VEO), Language Receptive Organization (LRO), and Language Expressive Organization (LEO). At the receptive level, processing that involves one modality (visual or auditory) is defined as *intrasensory* reception, and processing that involves two modalities (auditory *and* visual) is *intersensory* reception. This design provides assessment of visual, auditory, and auditory/visual reception and visual-motor and verbal expression, and fits nicely into the framework of Table 5.8; again, however, Basic Neurological Functions/Intactness (I), Gross Motor Expressive (III-C), and Mental Activity (IV-C) functions need supplementary evaluation.

- The Wechsler Preschool and Primary Scale of Intelligence-Revised (WPPSI-R; Wechsler, 1989) is applicable to children ages 3–7¼ years. As with the other Wechsler scales, a Verbal and a Performance IQ score are obtained. Each contains five core subtests and an optional subtest. For early childhood neuropsychological assessment, inclusion of the optional subtests *(animal pegs* [association of colors and symbols in a speeded fine-motor format] and *sentence memory*) is strongly recommended. No measure of Basic Neurological Functions/Intactness or Gross Motor Expressive functions is obtained on the WPPSI-R.

- The Stanford-Binet Fourth Edition (SB-4; Thorndike, Hagen, & Sattler, 1986) (applicable from ages 2 through adulthood) provides four area scores: (1) *verbal reasoning* (four subtests), (2) *quantitative reasoning* (three tasks), (3) *abstract/visual reasoning* (four subtests), and (4) *short-term memory* (four subtests). Theoretically, the first two areas are thought to measure *crystallized abilities*, whereas abstract/visual reasoning is considered to be a measure of *fluid-analytic intelligence*. Short-term memory is felt to be an independent function. Although this test has definite neuropsychological applications, the insufficient test floor in the age range of 4–5 years makes it difficult to detect mild to moderate problems. In addition, at younger ages, the number of subtests in any of the four areas is decreased, thereby limiting thorough assessment of certain functions (e.g., short-term memory). As is the case with many of the previous tests, neurological and gross motor functions are not evaluated.

- The Leiter International Performance Scale-Revised (Roid & Miller, 1997) contains 20 subtests that measure nonverbal intelligence. The first 10 subtests in the Primary Battery measure traditional intelligence constructs such as reasoning, visualization, and problem solving. The second 10 subtests in the Supplemental Battery measure attention and memory. A traditional IQ measure is derived from the Primary Battery. Items in the Primary Battery include measurement of figure-ground, form completion, matching, repeated patterns, classification, and sequential order. Supplementary Battery tests involve forward memory of object sequences, reverse memory, sustained attention, and immediate recognition of missing objects. Fluid (nonverbal) intelligence is assessed, and the Leiter-R was designed to evaluate children with motor impairments, communication disorders, hearing impairments, or certain types of learning disabilities. Although each battery takes 45–60 minutes, a shorter "Core Battery" (consisting of four subtests) provides a quick (20 minute) measure of intelligence. Because the Leiter-R is nonverbal and/or nonmotor, it has definite potential in evaluating children who have neuromotor handicaps.

SUMMARY

Early childhood neuropsychological assessment overlaps pediatric, developmental, and intelligence evaluations. Although some tests are specifically designed to assess neuropsychological function per se (e.g., NEPSY), others geared toward development or IQ still provide data that can be subject to neuropsychological interpretation. First-order interpretation of data should be on the subtest level, with secondary analysis being at a core or grouped-subtest level. In early childhood neuropsychology, use of summary indexes or aggregate scores is *not* recommended. Aggregate scores often obscure problems, as high scores on one subtest may cancel out low scores on another, perhaps leading to a summary score that appears "average." Description of areas of strength and weakness also moves toward more reliable qualitative information, a key element in infant and early childhood neuropsychology.

Further Assessment Considerations

In previous chapters, it was emphasized that infant and early childhood neuropsychology was transdisciplinary in nature. Given the shared emphasis on motor development, exploring approaches to infant motor assessment found in the occupational and physical therapy literature is logical (see Case-Smith, 1996 for a review).

The basic premise of *neuromaturational theory* is that the rate and sequence of motor development are essentially invariant in "normal" infants, and that motor skill maturation reflects the hierarchy of CNS development. More specifically, as the infant matures, higher cortical brain centers inhibit lower, reflexive brain centers such as the brain stem. More refined and coordinated movements are the result of increasing cortical control, and these abilities replace more immature, reflexive movement patterns.

In contrast, *contemporary dynamic systems theory* holds that perceptual input associated with movement cannot be separated from the movement it produces; perception and movement continually interact in learning. For example, visual, vestibular, and proprioceptive systems enable the infant to orient head and body for balance and ambulation. Similarly, grasping patterns are refined based on tactile and kinesthetic feedback in conjunction with visual input. Therefore, not only does perception guide action, but the infant's movement creates his or her perception of the world (Case-Smith, 1996). Multisensory input enters and travels through the CNS as a unit and is integrated at all levels, including at the receptor site. The infant derives meaning from the environment through a continuous stream of multisensory input; all learning is based on this integration of sensory information (Thelen, 1995).

Therefore, besides the integrated influence of the CNS, systems and experiences outside the CNS also have a strong influence on motor development.

Chapter 6

The infant's ability to adjust and vary motor activity in a flexible, smooth manner is considered the hallmark of normal movement. *Quality of movement* (Miller & Roid, 1994) therefore is critical in evaluation of neuromotor behavior, more so than static indicators such as achievement of milestones or ability to maintain positions. Documentation of the infant's ability to move from one posture to another or from one toy to another under a variety of conditions appears more important than the ability to achieve or maintain any one posture or movement. Coordinated *sequences* of movement are the basic unit of motor skill and the most essential components of motor evaluation (Case-Smith, 1996).

This approach reflects the interactive nature of neuromotor development, in which *intrinsic* (muscle bulk, strength, biomechanical constraints, perceptual abilities) and *extrinsic* (environmental factors such as the type of task the infant is faced with or the objects that are manipulated) form a reciprocal relationship. The emphasis on qualitative information, determination of the functional significance of a neuromotor deficit, and consideration of the transactional nature of the brain–behavior relationship all are prime tenets of infant and early childhood neuropsychology. Along neuropsychological lines, coordination of integrated, functional systems is considered more diagnostically useful because it reflects more complex, higher-order CNS synthesis. Therefore, observation of adaptability and how the infant learns new skills should also be a major consideration.

Clinicians and researchers involved in infant and early childhood neuropsychology should be aware of several new motor assessments that are based on dynamic systems theory. All measure functional movement in the infant's natural environment, and are flexible enough to obtain the infant's best performance. The instruments also measure qualitative aspects of posture and movement. By measuring individual components that define the quality of movement, they are sensitive to change or progress in motor performance (Case-Smith, 1996).

Alberta Infant Motor Scale (AIMS)

The AIMS (Piper & Darrah, 1994) is applicable in the assessment of motor maturation from 40 weeks gestational age through the age of independent walking. The test is *observational*, with minimal handling, and the motor sequences involved in the development of postural control in prone, sitting, supine, and standing are described. Motor patterns in activities such as rolling or transitioning into sitting or standing are rated, in addition to postures. The test is useful in infants who are at risk for motor delays and it identifies emerging and established skills. Items involve weight bearing and antigravity movement (vestibular and proprioceptive input). Even if the test is not employed in neuropsychological assessment per se, familiarity with the normal developmental sequences that are presented is recommended.

Toddler and Infant Movement Evaluation (TIME)

The TIME (Miller & Roid, 1994) is applicable to children from 4 to 42 months of age. A pictorial format is employed and parent participation is involved in test administration. There are three primary subtests: Mobility (supine, prone, sitting, standing, ambulating; these are scored from immature to mature moving in position), Stability (scored from observations made when administering the Mobility and Motor Organization Scales; different scores are assigned to items previously rated), and Social/Emotional Abilities (scored 1 [lowest] to 5 [highest], measuring state/activity level, attention, and emotions/reactions). In addition there are the Motor Organization (rated from the infant's behaviors during parent-elicited play) and Functional Performance subtests (series of questions regarding the child's adaptive behavior in areas of self-care, self-management, relationships, and community functioning). Optional tests include the Atypical Positions Subtest (24 positions that are indicative of motor delays or deviations), the Quality Rating Subtest (scored 1–4, with 4 being indicative of normal motor functioning), and the Component Analysis Subtest (to document small increments of change). The TIME is excellent in the diagnosis of motor delays and dysfunctions, in planning intervention, and in the evaluation of changes in motor performance resulting from intervention and maturation.

Posture and Fine Motor Assessment of Infants (PFMAI)

The PFMAI (Case-Smith & Bigsby, 1993) contains 36 items that measure posture (proximal stability, alignment, movement against gravity, and postural control) and 41 items that measure accuracy and quality of reach, grasping patterns, release, and control of arm and hand movements. The PFMAI is useful in the first year of life, and items are scored with flexibility and with minimal handling of the infant.

Test of Infant Motor Performance (TIMP)

The TIMP (Campbell, Kolobe, Osten, Girolami, & Lenki, 1994) was designed to evaluate postural control and movement in infants, 32 weeks gestational age through 4 months. The test contains two scales: (1) the elicited scale, which rates the infant's ability to display coordinated postural responses when placed in a variety of spatial orientations (e.g., rolling, pull-to-sit), and (2) the observed scale, rating the infant's spontaneous changes in positions, and orientation of the head and trunk (e.g., reaches for person or object, head lift in prone).

Peabody Developmental Motor Scales

The Peabody Developmental Motor Scales (Folio & Fewell, 1983) is not based on dynamic systems theory, but allows for *norm-referenced evaluation* of gross (170 items) and fine motor (112 items) development in children from birth to 83 months of age. The gross motor scale involves reflexes, balance, nonlocomotor, locomotor, and "receipt and propulsion" (rolling a ball, kicking a ball). The fine motor scale involves grasping, hand use, eye–hand coordination, and manual dexterity. Items are scored on a three-point scale, and although this affords more detailed evaluation than does the Bayley Scales, this test does not measure qualitative aspects of motor performance.

Summary

In summary, the bulk of tests listed above tap movement patterns, these being good indicators of the infant's ability to integrate multisensory information. Most are observational, naturalistic, and employ parents and use of toys. Except for the Peabody, these tests also evaluate patterns of movement or "synergies," rather than singular motor acts or motor milestones, and the quality and adaptability of movement patterns. Absence of adaptability or limited flexibility in motor patterns is considered indicative of motor dysfunction, particularly if either is found on repeated assessment over time. In reference to early neuropsychological theory, the ability to integrate multisensory information and transition from one posture to another incorporates *integrated functional systems.* The infant's ability to integrate and adapt the coordination of functional systems in response to altered sensory input and environmental demands is an excellent indicator of overall CNS intactness and potential.

DIAGNOSTIC INDICATORS

In assessing abnormalities, a firm foundation in normal development is necessary. Clinicians need to consider that all babies are different, and some are simply temporarily slow in their development. However, the further away from "average" in a particular skill a baby is, the more likely he or she is abnormal. Moreover, *combinations* or *clusters* of findings are important (Egan, Illingworth, & MacKeith, 1976; Ellenberg & Nelson, 1988).

> **Case 1.** M. J. is a 12-month-old girl, born at term, who has a very small head circumference (>1½ SDs below average for height and weight). When given the BINS, she scores in the low-risk range. In

contrast, B.A. is a 12-month-old girl, also born at term, who has an equally small head circumference, but who scores in the high-risk range on the BINS.

This example underscores an important point, namely, that in B.A.'s case, the abnormal finding of a small head circumference in conjunction with other indicators (high-risk score on the BINS) is of more concern than M.J.'s small head circumference in isolation. Although continued monitoring is warranted in the former situation, further investigation is necessary in the latter. Also, the longer an abnormal finding persists, the more likely it is to be clinically significant.

Therefore, interpretation of dysfunction depends on: (1) the particular abnormality or abnormalities that are found, (2) the presence of a constellation of abnormal findings, and (3) the abnormal signs in conjunction with a history of risk factors (Egan et al., 1976).

Another major premise in detection of abnormality involves the structure–function relationship alluded to earlier (e.g., Prechtl, 1984). Growth and differentiation of the CNS does not consist of a simple, predetermined "readout" of genetic programs, but involves an interaction with extrinsic factors in an extremely complex epigenetic process. The interaction between structure and function becomes intricate and function may: (1) speed up regressive cell death at the neuronal and synaptic level, (2) be needed by neural structures for their own maintenance (e.g., cortical representation of the visual system), (3) when changed from normal, alter feedback and transiently or even permanently change connectivity (Prechtl, 1984). Moreover, there is continuity from prenatal to postnatal life with the motor patterns of the fetus and premature infant becoming linked to specific stimulus conditions to which the infant is exposed after birth. Stated differently, reflexive motor patterns are present early on, but then are applied to extrinsic situations. The interaction between the pattern and the situation will shape subsequent neural organization. This fact underscores why environmental stimulation is critical at early ages.

Administration of various neuropsychological instruments provides examiners the opportunity to detect pathognomonic indicators during the evaluation session. Many of these are not the result of maturational lags, but are indicative of abnormal development or neurological impairment (Aylward, 1995). Items can be considered *neurodevelopmental* (tone, posture, movement) or *neurobehavioral* (visual tracking, auditory orientation, alertness, cry).

Amiel-Tison (1976) classified biologically at-risk infants, evaluated over the first year, into three typical patterns: (1) normal, (2) transitory anomalies with normalization by the end of the first year, and (3) signs of definitive brain damage. With transitory anomalies, two patterns emerge: in the first 3 months there is (a) irritability, global hypertonia, or hypertonia in the neck extensors or (b) lethargy and global hypotonia. Improvement in these patterns becomes observable at around 3 months. However, from 3 to 9 months there is irritability, persistent flexor tone in lower limbs, poor active tone in neck and trunk, and hyperreflexivity. Normalization of these signs is observed around 9 months, or there may be transitory spastic hemiplegia. Definitive brain damage includes hydrocephaly, microcephaly, hypotonia, tetraplegia or seizure disorder. *Spastic hemiplegia* (involving one side of the body) or *diplegia* (lower extremities) are diagnosed by 9 months.

Indicators of *hemiplegia* are not easily found prior to 6 months in infants with documented, unilateral hemispheric lesions. Signs become more obvious between 6 and 12 months, and deterioration of existing skills can also occur. In general, the earlier the signs of neurodevelopmental dysfunction, the more severe is the hemiplegia (Bouza, Rutherford, Acolet, Pennock, & Dubowitz, 1994).

Prechtl (1977) delineated three *syndromes of abnormality* that are found in the newborn period:

- *Hyperexcitable*: low-frequency, high-amplitude tremors, increased intensity of tendon reflexes, low-threshold Moro response, with associated increased resistance against passive movements, prolonged crying, hyperkinesis, and instability of states.
- *Apathetic*: low intensity and high threshold for responses, many responses absent, decreased resistance against passive movements, hypokinesis, and difficult to rouse (hemisyndrome often is present afterwards).
- *Comatose*: slow or abnormal responses, absent or weak arousal to various stimuli (including pain and vestibular stimulation).

In both of these classification schemas, the presence of syndromes or groupings of findings is diagnostically and prognostically significant.

Neurobehavioral Indicators

> **Case 2.** M. L. is a 3-year-old boy, born at 26 weeks gestational age. When evaluated at 6 months, he was noted to have jerky eye movements, and he would not focus on small objects such as a pellet. He presently is doing very poorly on perceptual-performance tasks on the Differential Ability Scales or the McCarthy Scales of Children's Abilities. M. L.'s referring physician questions whether there is a connection between the earlier findings and the current test results.

This case underscores the fact that whenever visual items are administered to infants, examiners should pay particular attention to deviations in gaze, aberrant eye positioning, or uncoordinated eye movement. Concerning positioning, the *setting sun sign* (downward eye deviation with paresis of upward gaze, retraction of the upper eyelid, and exposed sclera over the rim of the iris) indicates increased intracranial pressure (Baird & Gordon, 1983). *Nystagmus* is involuntary, rhythmical, conjugate oscillatory eye movements that can be slow (pendular) or jerky, and may be secondary to a variety of ophthalmological and neurological conditions (CNS, eye, inner ear). *Strabismus* is a condition in which the eyes are not maintained parallel, with one or both eyes deviating inward (esotropia) or outward (exotropia). Infants should also be able to track horizontally and vertically by 2 months, followed by circular tracking by 3 months.

Excessive irritability or a *high-pitched cry* are significant findings, as is overreactivity or underreactivity to auditory input (including orientation to auditory stimuli). Decreased alertness, lack of awareness of surroundings, and impaired social interactive abilities are other significant indicators.

Neurodevelopmental Indicators

> **Case 3.** R. K. was noted to be very floppy at 3–4 months of age. At 6 months, poor coordination and an increase in tone were found. By 9–10 months, he seemed very "tight," particularly in the legs. His parents have been told that R. K. has cerebral palsy and they are questioning the developmental neuropsychologist as to whether their son is actually getting "worse."

With regard to muscle tone, bilateral use of the upper and lower extremities should always be present, as should symmetrical muscle tone and movement (equal on both sides of the body). *Hypotonia* (decreased muscle tone) is one of the most frequent early abnormal signs, often being caused by: (1) CNS, (2) metabolic, or (3) neuromuscular disorders (Aicardi & Bax, 1992). Many children who display early hypotonia improve. In fact, there is a general improvement in tone abnormalities (hyper- and hypotonia) over the first 18–24 months (Ellenberg & Nelson, 1988; Georgieff, Bernbaum, Hoffman-Williamson, & Daft, 1986). The prevalence of abnormal tone, particularly *hypertonia* (increased tone) is highest at 3–4 months and decreases thereafter. A syndrome known as *transient hypertonicity* or *transient neurological signs of prematurity* may occur in up to 50% of VLBW infants. It is characterized by hypertonicity, reflex abnormalities, back and neck arching, shoulder retraction, motor delays, and irritability. These abnormal signs improve significantly or disappear by 12 months of age.

Persistent, abnormal muscle function is typically termed *cerebral palsy* (CP). This disorder is heterogeneous, and may be manifest in abnormalities of tone, movement, or posture, and is sometimes only evident when a child is engaged in activities that involve coordination or regulation of muscle tone. The disorder begins early in life and is *not* the result of underlying progressive disease. CP can be classified as *spastic* (e.g., hemiplegia, diplegia, tetraplegia, paraplegia), *dyskinetic* (athetosis, dystonia), *hypotonic* (atonic diplegia, hypotonia, and ataxia), *ataxic*, and *mixed* (e.g., spasticity and ataxia). Pathognomonic indicators may surface as an inability to restrict movements to an intended pattern or location. Examples include a cortical thumb sign (in which the hands are fisted with the thumb appearing to be grasped by the fingers), motor overflow, or tremors. Many children first displaying hypotonia at 6–12 weeks of age followed by a *dystonic* stage (poor quality of movement and diffuse increase in tone) are subsequently diagnosed with CP. At 8 to 9 months, the child becomes spastic, with a predominance of hip and knee flexor positioning (Aicardi & Bax, 1992). *Spastic diplegia* (symmetric, bilateral lower extremity hypertonicity) and *spastic hemiplegia* (hypertonicity on one side of the body) can be detected by 9 months of age, but is often not diagnosed until the infant is 18–24 months old (Harris, 1991). Premature infants account for two-thirds of all cases of spastic diplegia and one-fourth to one-third of all cases of hemiplegia. *Quadriplegic CP* (abnormal tone of all four extremities with involvement of the head and trunk) is more obvious and detection occurs earlier, with the mean age being 5 months (Harris, 1991). Examiners should be aware that transient increased tone in the lower extremities is found frequently in infants born prematurely and improves between 6 and 12 months of age (Georgieff et al., 1986). This has been referred to as *transient dystonia* (Drillien, 1972).

Spastic diplegia is more frequent in preterm infants because the areas of the premature infant's brain most vulnerable to injury are to the sides of the lateral ventricles, where fibers from the motor cortex travel through the internal capsule down to the limbs. Fibers to the legs are medial, and fibers to the arms are more lateral.

In addition, persistence of primitive reflexes (Moro, asymmetric tonic neck reflex [ATNR]) and absence of postural reactions (e.g., parachute) by 2 years of age are associated with a poor prognosis for ambulation (Sala & Grant, 1995).

Some infants and children appear to "outgrow" CP (Piper, Mazur, Silver, & Ramsay, 1988), as muscle tone abnormalities can resolve over the first 2 years of life. However, an increased likelihood of later high-prevalence/low-severity dysfunctions is present in these children (Drillien, 1972). As many as two-thirds of infants who display hypertonia subsequently have speech/language, fine motor/adaptive, and behavior problems at 2–3 years of age. At 5 years, one-fourth display learning disabilities, language problems, perceptual dysfunctions, and hyperactivity/attention deficits.

Clinicians should be aware of the fact that slow, smooth, passive movement will produce less resistance in a spastic extremity than will fast movement.

However, the response in a child with normal muscle tone is consistent, regardless of speed, unless resistance is voluntary (Baird & Gordon, 1983). Also, awareness of the reflex grading scheme used by physicians is important. A response such as the patellar reflex (knee jerk) is graded:

- 0 = absent
- +/- = very faint or trace
- 1+ = hypoactive
- 2+ = normal
- 3+ = hyperactive
- 4+ = hyperactive with clonus

Although infant and early childhood neuropsychologists should be careful not to overstep diagnostic boundaries with physical or neurological diagnoses, careful observation of a variety of aspects of the child's function is definitely within the purview of this discipline. For example, observation of the method of ambulation is important in early childhood neuropsychology. Mechanisms used in standing must be integrated with the walking sequence. An abnormal gait in toddlers and older children could be the result of various neurological and orthopedic abnormalities. Definitions of abnormal gait include:

1	*Ataxic gait* characterized by unsteady, uncoordinated, wide-based method of walking (often more pronounced with the eyes closed). There is irregular staggering to either side, lurching or swaying forward or backward. Walking on a line is particularly difficult, and this gait can resemble a person with alcohol intoxication.
2	*Spastic hemiplegic gait* is characterized by toe walking secondary to contracture of the Achilles tendon, with subsequent equinus posturing of the foot which essentially makes the limb functionally longer on the affected side. The child arcs the leg away from the hip (*circumduction*), or compensates by tilting the pelvis upward and dragging the foot (toe).
3	*Spastic diplegic gait* is characterized by bilateral toe walking with hip and knee flexion, resulting in walking with a stiff, shuffling gait and abduction of the lower extremities so that the knees bump one another, in a crouched position. One foot crosses in front of the other in a scissors gait.
4	*Dystonia* and *athetosis (extrapyramidal gait)* involve irregular writhing contortions of the proximal hip muscles and trunk and neck. There may be a tendency to throw the head backwards (or from side to side), grimacing of the face, and unusual movements of the extremities. The posture of the trunk and body can change rapidly.

> 5 | *Muscular dystrophy* is characterized by profound hip weakness, resulting in thoraco-lumbar lordosis and an exaggerated rotation of the pelvis, throwing the hips from side to side as weight shifts with each step in a waddling type of movement (Baird & Gordon, 1983).

Similarly, observation of the upper extremity movement is also important. However, in infancy and early childhood, many so-called soft signs are of limited diagnostic utility. For example, although *synkinesia* (presence of abnormal mirror movements or overflow of fine finger movement from one hand to the other) is suggestive of problems if it is exaggerated, *dysdiadochokinesia* (ability to perform rapid alternating movements such as rapid pronation and supination of the hand) or *graphesthesia* (ability to recognize a number by feel when the number is traced on the palm of the hand) and *stereognosis* are not reliable findings in this age range. Also, from age 2 onwards hand preference becomes established, although infants and young preschoolers are still somewhat ambidextrous. By age 3–4½ laterality becomes definite; strong or exclusive use of one hand or foot in the very young child (under 2 years of age) is considered to be abnormal.

Interestingly, Saigal, Rosenbaum, Szatmari, and Hoult (1992) found that the proportion of left-handedness was significantly higher in a cohort of ELBW children (born < 1000 g) at 8 years of age than in control infants who were born at term. These authors suggested an association between neurological impairment and non-right-handedness, and others have indicated associations between left-handedness, ambidexterity, and cognitive and behavioral deficits. Therefore, in at least a proportion of biologically at-risk infants, non-right-handedness has a pathological basis (Powls, Botting, Cooke, & Marlow, 1996). However, finger movements and finger postures are not felt to be a good indicator of brain damage in preterm infants because of the wide overlap between the performance of normal and brain-damaged young infants (Konishi & Prechtl, 1994).

Observation can also include physical findings such as abnormalities in head circumference or stature, or dysmorphic features of the head and skull, face (eyes, nose, mouth, ears), neck, limbs, digits, or skin and hair.

Abnormal movements (characteristic of extrapyramidal dysfunction) include:

> 1 | *Myoclonus* (quick, unpredictable, nonrhythmic contraction of single muscles or small muscle groups, resulting in a sudden, jerky movement of the limb), which often is seen in newborns but is significant if persistent past the age of 3 months

2	*Tremor* (involuntary, rhythmic trembling or quivering) which can be static (at rest) or with intention (induced by voluntary activity), and often is related to basal ganglia dysfunction
3	*Chorea* and *athetosis* (the former being rapid, involuntary jerks, the latter, slow, "wormlike" repetitive movements); both can be increased with attempted activity, emotional stress, or sensory stimulation
4	*Dystonic movements* (sudden muscular spasms, primarily involving neck and trunk muscles)

Prechtl, Ferrari, and Cioni (1993) reported that perinatal asphyxia has important effects on the spontaneous motility of asphyxiated, full-term infants. Hypokinesis occurred frequently during the first days of life, followed by a transient or prolonged (> 15 to 22 weeks) abnormal quality of general movements.

Several early pathognomonic indicators have repeatedly been associated with increased risk for later problems. These include:

- Neck extensor hypertonia (with shoulder elevation and retraction, and brisk deep tendon reflexes)
- Truncal tone hypertonicity
- Poor visual attention/following
- Lack of midline behaviors
- Inability to sit supported with head erect (by 4 months)
- Inability to bear weight on forearms when prone (by 3 months)
- Hands always fisted (after 3 months)
- Asymmetries in posture
- Hyperexcitability
- Pull-to-stand instead of pull-to-sit (5–6 months)
- Presence of early hypertonicity (by 4 months)
- Asymmetric tonic neck posturing (fencing posture) that persists past 6 months

Neuromotor problems can be found in children whose other areas of development are essentially normal. Moreover, higher cortical function can still remain intact despite extensive brain damage (Baird & Gordon, 1983). The diagnostic and predictive power of abnormal physical findings improves with an increasing number of these findings, in conjunction with the child's failure to meet motor milestones. Along the lines of the issue of *functional significance*, if a child passes all motor milestones but has some abnormal physical findings (e.g., tightness of the heel cords), the likelihood of later neurodevelopmental problems is decreased. The combination of pathognomonic findings with delays in developmental milestones warrants more detailed neurological and developmental assessment.

Finally, there are certain assessment mistakes that must be avoided. These include the following:

1	Failure to base diagnostic opinion on examination of the child as a whole (including consistency between the history and current findings)
2	Failure to recognize artificially depressed performance secondary to illness, hunger, or fatigue at the time of testing
3	Making a diagnosis based on single items, versus a combination of items
4	Failure to recognize individual variation (including familial traits, slow maturation), and failure to consider all factors that may have affected development, including illness, drugs, environment, and early CNS insults (Illingworth, 1990)

Perhaps one of the most critical mistakes that can be made in early developmental neuropsychology or any assessment, is to assume that poor performance or an inability to successfully complete a task is the result of intrinsic limitations, whereas in actuality the limitations are the result of extrinsic constraints.

Directions

The focus of this volume has been on neuropsychological and neurodevelopmental assessment. However, clinicians should realize that electrophysiological correlates such as auditory evoked responses (AER) and visual evoked responses (VER) also hold promise as diagnostic and predictive neuropsychological techniques, either used individually or with neurobehavioral measures (e.g., D. Molfese, 1992; D. L. Molfese & Molfese, 1979, 1986). Similarly, *visual habituation/recognition memory* (Fagan & Detterman, 1992; Fagan & Singer, 1983) is a useful technique that has application in early developmental neuropsychological assessment. Unfortunately, space limitations and the *clinical* nature of this book preclude elaboration of these techniques, and their absence is not meant to reflect negatively on their merit. Use of these techniques in conjunction with neurodevelopmental measures such as the BINS (Aylward, 1995) in the prediction of later outcome would be a fertile area of research.

NEW DIRECTIONS FOR ASSESSMENT

Neuroimaging techniques (CT, MRI) and functional neuroimaging procedures (PET, SPECT, and echoplanar MRI [functional MRI]) (Havey, 1995) hold promise in applications to infant and early childhood neuropsychology. However, these techniques are not widely available because of the cost and procedural requirements necessary to maintain the machinery (cyclotron) and most likely would be employed at a research, versus applied, level.

Functional imaging methods involving noninvasive FMRI and minimally invasive SPECT and PET enable the investigation of brain abnormality and neuropathology. Cerebral blood flow (PET or SPECT), oxygen or glucose metabolism (PET), and functional activity of the brain (FMRI) would be particularly useful in evaluation of early neuropsychological dysfunctions and recovery from CNS insults. Echoplanar MRI is probably the wave of the future in this regard (see Anderson & Gore, 1997; Giedd, 1997). EEGs and ultrasound also have a role in developmental neuropsychology, as do VERs and brain electrical activity mapping (BEAM), which combines both EEG and evoked responses. In fact, because of these imaging techniques, identification of the type and location of a lesion is not as important in infant and early childhood neuropsychology. Instead, the focus of testing is to determine the functional capabilities of the child (Stoddart & Knight, 1986).

Much remains to be done in the area of neurobehavioral/neuropsychological assessment. Batchelor (1996), in reference to pediatric neuropsychology, wrote, "The pediatric neuropsychologist requires extensive knowledge of the relationship between central nervous system development (including cerebral organization, laterality, and plasticity) and the emergence of cognitive functions from birth through early adulthood" (p. 10). Understanding these relationships is a prerequisite for the proper selection and administration of assessments and interpretation of data that are obtained. Without doubt, these requirements are equally critical, yet even more complex, in infant and early childhood neuropsychology.

There continues to be a need for assessment techniques based on neuropsychological frameworks that span the infant through early childhood age range in a continuous fashion. For example, a bridging test is needed that would connect the BINS (Aylward, 1995) and the FirstSTEP (Miller, 1993) between 2 and 3 years. Moreover, the relationships between neonatal tests such as the Neurobehavioral Assessment of the Preterm Infant (NAPI; Korner & Thom, 1990) or the Brief Infant Neurobehavioral Optimality Scale (Aylward, Verhulst, & Colliver, 1985) and later tests such as the BINS or ENORS (Aylward, 1994) need to be investigated further.

Various conceptual issues need clarification. A major problem is translating the qualitative information obtained from infant and early childhood neuropsychological testing into more objective, quantifiable data. The *optimality approach* offers some advantages, but has not been applied to early childhood assessment. Presently, many functions are linked with test items in a post hoc manner, rather than defining a function and devising a task to assess it. Therefore, development of tests with underlying neuropsychological frameworks is necessary.

Data interpretation also becomes more difficult because major premises of later neuropsychological evaluation such as laterality or executive functions are not as applicable at younger ages. For example, from middle childhood onwards, if verbal functioning is lower than nonverbal functioning, it is assumed that the child suffers from left hemispheric dysfunction (e.g., verbal IQ < performance IQ); conversely, if nonverbal functioning is poorer than verbal abilities (VIQ > PIQ), then the possibility of right hemispheric problems is more likely. If there is no distinct pattern of weakness, with both areas being equally affected, then both hemispheres are assumed to be dysfunctional. Laterality findings must be tempered in infants and young children. This caveat is made in light of findings that words are processed better via the right ear from age 4 onwards, face recognition is better when processed through the left visual field from age 6, and grip strength and finger tapping are stronger and more efficient on the right between 3 and 5 years of age. In fact, the IQ of children with right hemispheric lesions tends to be lower than in those with lesions of the left hemisphere (where the FSIQ is minimally depressed) (Nass & Stiles, 1996).

Another major dilemma faced in this type of assessment is that the probability of detecting subtle damage is greater with increased age, because of the enhanced sophistication of later assessment instruments. However, the longer the time interval between the insult and an assessment, the greater is the influence of intervening variables, particularly the environment. Therefore, earlier assessment has a better potential to explain potential cause-and-effect relationships, although there are limitations on exactly what can be assessed. At later ages, assessment techniques are better, but cause-and-effect relationships are more muddled, largely because of environmental influences and plasticity (Aylward, 1988). Thus, development of more accurate predictive models of dysfunction is another area needing emphasis in infant and early childhood neuropsychology.

A prime focus of later neuropsychological assessment is to differentiate abnormal and normal functioning. However, the boundaries of normality are less clear in infancy and early childhood, which makes such a differentiation more difficult. It is recommended that combinations of pathognomonic signs *and* patterns of performance must be considered at younger ages.

It is also more difficult to complete lengthy evaluations with infants and young children because of fatigue, irritability, and normally short attention spans. As a result, neuropsychological screening instruments are needed more at this age than at any other. This is particularly the case in large-volume clinics, and in light of decreasing reimbursement opportunities and the costs inherent in more lengthy tests. In addition, development of neurodevelopmental/neuropsychological prescreening methods such as parent questionnaires should be pursued. Prescreening would allow neuropsychological "evaluation" techniques to be applied to greater numbers of children, and become more routine in pediatric care. More detailed assessment could then be reserved for infants and young children who demonstrated problems on the prescreening.

The purpose of infant and early childhood evaluation needs to be clearly defined. Early assessment: (1) provides information on the child's current status, (2) identifies children who would benefit from intervention (Aylward, 1996), and (3) also affords predictive utility. Moreover, evaluation may have clinical, research, or combined applications. The purpose of the assessment will determine the type and breadth of evaluation employed. For example, if the main purpose of early neuropsychological evaluation is to identify children at biological risk who should receive early intervention, then a screening instrument may suffice.

If the neuropsychologist is more interested in identification of subtle areas of dysfunction that may result from application of innovative medical procedures or in utero exposure to drugs, then more detailed evaluation may be necessary for research purposes. Regardless of the purpose, these evaluations should not be administered by psychometric technicians who are not trained in early developmental neuropsychology. Another area that needs further exploration involves the relationship between the initial assessment performance and the influence of intervention on subsequent assessment performance (V. J. Molfese, 1992). Similarly, linkages between early and later assessment findings are necessary.

TRAINING ISSUES

Early developmental neuropsychology requires specific training that is not routinely available in traditional clinical or developmental psychology programs (Aylward, 1988). In addition to specialized psychology coursework, training should be closely allied to pediatrics, pediatric neurology, neonatology, genetics, occupational and physical therapy, and interdisciplinary clinics. Presently, because of limited training opportunities, the "newness" of the subspecialty, and vagaries and absence of a clear definition, a lack of acceptance is fostered in psychology and other disciplines, including medicine. However, a significant component of early developmental neuropsychological assessment is behavioral observation, and psychologists are specialists in the observation of behavior. Therefore, a key point in early developmental neuropsychology is to make examiners better versed in which behaviors to elicit and to observe (Aylward, 1988).

Core coursework recommendations for a specialty in neuropsychology have been forwarded by a combined committee of the International Neuropsychological Society and Division 40 of the American Psychological Association (reprinted in Hynd & Willis, 1988). However, these recommendations are not totally applicable to early developmental neuropsychology. Drotar and Sturm (1989) also offered recommendations regarding training psychologists as "*infant specialists.*" They stated that "competency as a psychologist/infant specialist is achieved through didactic and clinical training with specialized infant populations under close supervision" (p. 58). Interestingly, many of the roles of the infant specialist are identical to those of the early developmental neuropsychologist, including assessment of infant cognitive development, clinical interventions with caretakers, direct interventions with infants, consultation and collaboration with other professionals, and research. Consideration of the interdependence of cognitive, sensorimotor, and socioemotional development and environmental issues is also critical (Drotar & Sturm, 1989).

Several types of clinical training programs could be altered to fit the early developmental neuropsychological model. These are programs in clinical child, applied developmental, pediatric, and school psychology. Moreover, clinical and research training in infant and early childhood neuropsychology can also occur at the practicum, graduate, internship or postdoctoral level.

Drawing on the suggestions of Hynd and Willis (1988), Drotar and Sturm (1989), and Aylward (1988, 1994), the following curriculum recommendations are forwarded.

Core Courses

1	Child development
2	Developmental psychology
3	Tests and measurement
4	Statistics and methodology
5	Perception
6	Physiological
7	Family development
8	Infancy

Clinical Courses

1	Child psychopathology
2	Intelligence testing
3	Developmental testing
4	Interviewing
5	Behavior therapy/modification
6	Psychotherapy
7	Exceptional child

Basic Neuroscience

1	Advanced physiological
2	Psychopharmacology
3	Neurobiology
4	Developmental neuroanatomy
5	Research design in neuropsychology
6	Clinical neurology/neuropathology
7	Specialized neurodevelopmental assessment techniques

Practica/Internships ━━

■ *Populations/clinics:* high-risk infants, infants with mental retardation, developmental disabilities, physical handicaps, chronic illnesses, language/communication disorders or neurobehavioral disorders, pediatric neurology clinics, genetics clinics, neonatal intensive care units, normal newborn nurseries, infant and preschool day-care centers, school early childhood screening clinics, multidisciplinary specialty and diagnostic clinics.

■ *Experiences:* assessment, intervention (different ages, different dysfunctions), observation, treatment planning, environmental assessment, parent interviewing/feedback, behavior therapy, consultation and liaison, interdisciplinary team participation, naturalistic assessment, interdisciplinary research, anticipatory guidance.

■ *Collaborations:* pediatrics, child psychiatry, pediatric neurology, developmental/behavioral pediatrics, pediatric rehabilitation, occupational/physical therapy, genetics, pediatric neurology, neonatology, early intervention, special education, speech/language pathology.

Training should occur with members of other disciplines, and a broad experience is necessary to familiarize the clinician with the clinical problems and assessment techniques.

The literature base should be broadened as well. In addition to the usual psychology journals, clinicians and researchers in early developmental neuropsychology would be well advised to regularly peruse other journals including (but not limited to): *Developmental Medicine and Child Neurology, Early Human Development, Infant Behavior and Development, Infants and Young Children, Journal of Developmental and Behavioral Pediatrics, Developmental Neuropsychology, Seminars in Pediatric Neurology, Neuropediatrics,* and other pediatric, perinatal, and neurology journals.

Finally, a definite need in this area is for several *specialized centers of training* (Aylward, 1994). These centers should be psychology-based, and affiliated with medical facilities so as to provide the proper patient populations and participation from medical specialties. These centers should be strongly allied with applied developmental and child clinical/pediatric psychology programs, and could offer varying levels of training including coursework, practica, internships, and fellowships. Establishment of centers would be a major step in the emergence of infant and early childhood neuropsychology as a true specialty area.

References

Aicardi, J. (1992). *Diseases of the nervous system in childhood. Clinics in Developmental Medicine, No. 115/118.* London: Cambridge University Press.

Aicardi, J., & Bax, M. (1992). Cerebral palsy. In J. Aicardi (Ed.), *Diseases of the nervous system in childhood* (pp. 300–375). London: MacKeith Press.

Allen, M. C., & Capute, A. J. (1989). Neonatal neurodevelopmental examination as a predictor of neuromotor outcome in premature infants. *Pediatrics, 83,* 498–506.

Allen, M. C., Donohue, P. K., & Dusman, A. E. (1993). The limit of viability—Neonatal outcome of infants born at 22 to 25 weeks' gestation. *New England Journal of Medicine, 329,* 1597–1601.

Als, H., Lester, B., Tronick, E., & Brazelton, B. (1982). Toward a research instrument for the Assessment of Preterm Infants' Behavior (APIB). In H. Fitzgerald, B. Lester, & M. Yogman (Eds.), *Theory and research in behavioral pediatrics* (Vol. 1). New York: Plenum Press.

American Academy of Pediatrics, Committee on Fetus and Newborn. (1996). Use and abuse of the Apgar Score. *Pediatrics, 98,* 141–142.

Amiel-Tison, C. (1976). A method for neurologic evaluation within the first year of life. In L. Gluck (Ed.), *Current problems in pediatrics* (pp. 3–50). Chicago: Year Book Medical.

Amiel-Tison, C. (1982). Neurologic signs, aetiology, and implications. In P. Stratton (Ed.), *Psychology of the human newborn* (pp. 75–94). New York: Wiley.

Amiel-Tison, C., Banier, G., Shnider, S., Levinson, G., Hughes, S., & Stefani, S. (1982). A new neurologic and adaptive capacity scoring system for evaluating obstetric medications in fullterm newborns. *Anesthesiology, 56,* 340–350.

Amiel-Tison, C., & Grenier, A. (1986). *Neurological assessment during the first year of life.* New York: Oxford University Press.

Anastasiow, N. J. (1990). Implications of the neurobiological model for early intervention. In S. J. Meisels & J. P. Shonkoff (Eds.), *Handbook of early childhood intervention* (pp. 196–216). London: Cambridge University Press.

Anderson, A. W., & Gore, J. C. (1997). The physical basis of neuroimaging techniques. In B. S. Peterson (Ed.), *Neuroimaging. Child and Adolescent Psychiatric Clinics of North America, 6,* 213–264.

Andre-Thomas, Chesni, Y., & Saint-Anne Dargassies. (1960). *The neurological examination of the infant.* Little Club Clinics in Developmental Medicine, No. 1. London: National Spastics Society.

Apgar, V. (1953). A proposal for a new method of evaluation of the newborn infant. *Current Research in Anesthesia and Analgesia, 32,* 260–267.

Apgar, V., Holaday, D. A., James, L. S., Weisbrot, I. M., & Berrien, C. (1958). Evaluation of the newborn infant: Second report. *Journal of the American Medical Association, 168,* 1985–1988.

Aylward, G. P. (1981). The developmental course of behavioral states in preterm infants: A descriptive study. *Child Development, 52,* 564–568.

Aylward, G. P. (1982). Methadone outcome studies: Is it the methadone? *Journal of Pediatrics, 101,* 214–215.

Aylward, G. P. (1988). Infant and early childhood assessment. In M. Tramontana & S. Hooper (Eds.), *Assessment issues in child neuropsychology* (pp. 225–248). New York: Plenum Press.

Aylward, G. P. (1990). Environmental influences on developmental outcome of children at risk. *Infants and Young Children, 2,* 1–9.

Aylward, G. P. (1992). The relationship between environmental risk and developmental outcome. *Journal of Developmental and Behavioral Pediatrics, 13,* 222–229.

Aylward, G. P. (1993). Perinatal asphyxia: Effects of biologic and environmental risks. *Clinics in Perinatology, 20,* 433–449.

Aylward, G. P. (1994). Update on early developmental neuropsychologic assessment: The Early Neuropsychologic Optimality Rating Scales (ENORS). In M. G. Tramontana & S. R. Hooper (Eds.), *Advances in child neuropsychology* (Vol. 2, pp. 172–200). Berlin: Springer-Verlag.

Aylward, G. P. (1995). *The Bayley Infant Neurodevelopmental Screener manual.* San Antonio: The Psychological Corporation.

Aylward, G. P. (1996). Environmental risk, intervention and developmental outcome. *Ambulatory Child Health, 2,* 161–170.

Aylward, G. P., & Brown, J. (1974). *The Prechtl neurological examination with revisions for the developmental assessment of premature infants.* Atlanta: Grady Memorial Hospital.

Aylward, G. P., Dunteman, G., Hatcher, R. P., Gustafson, N., & Widmayer, S. (1985). The SES-Composite Index: A tool for developmental outcome studies. *Psychological Documents, 15* (Ms. No. 2682).

Aylward, G. P., Gustafson, N., Verhulst, S. J., & Colliver, J. A. (1987). Consistency in the diagnosis of cognitive, motor, and neurologic function over the first three years. *Journal of Pediatric Psychology, 12,* 77–98.

Aylward, G. P., & Kenny, T. J. (1979). Developmental follow-up: Inherent problems and a conceptual model. *Journal of Pediatric Psychology, 4,* 331–343.

Aylward, G. P., & Pfeiffer, S. I. (1991). Perinatal complications and cognitive neuropsychological outcome. In J. W. Gray & R. S. Dean (Eds.), *Neuropsychology of perinatal complications* (pp. 128–160). New York: Springer.

Aylward, G. P., Verhulst, S. J., & Bell, S. (1988a). The Early Neuropsychologic Optimality Rating Scale (ENORS-9): A new developmental follow-up technique. *Journal of Developmental and Behavioral Pediatrics, 9,* 140–146.

Aylward, G. P., Verhulst, S. J., & Bell, S. (1988b). The Eighteen Month Early Neuropsychologic Optimality Rating Scale (ENORS-18): A predictive assessment instrument. *Developmental Neuropsychology, 4,* 47–61.

Aylward, G. P., Verhulst, S. J., & Bell, S. (1989). Correlation of asphyxia, other risk factors and outcome. A contemporary view. *Developmental Medicine and Child Neurology, 31,* 329–340.

Aylward, G. P., Verhulst, S. J., & Bell, S. (1992). Predictive utility of the 24-month Early Neuropsychologic Optimality Rating Scale (ENORS-24). *Developmental Medicine and Child Neurology, 30*(Suppl. 66), 33–34.

Aylward, G. P., Verhulst, S. J., & Bell, S. (1994). Enhanced prediction of later "normal" outcome using infant neuropsychological assessment. *Developmental Neuropsychology, 10,* 377–394.

Aylward, G. P., Verhulst, S. J., & Bell, S. (1996). Predictive utility of the Bayley Infant Neurodevelopmental Screener (BINS) risk status classifications. *Developmental Medicine and Child Neurology, 38*(Suppl. 74), 26.

Aylward, G. P., Verhulst, S. J., & Colliver, J. A. (1985). Development of a brief infant neurobehavioral optimality scale: Longitudinal sensitivity and specificity. *Developmental Neuropsychology, 1,* 265–276.

Azzarelli, B., Caldemeyer, R. S., Phillips, J. P., & De Meyer, W. E. (1996). Hypoxic-ischemic encephalopathy in areas of primary myelination: A neuroimaging and PET study. *Pediatric Neurology, 14*, 108–116.

Baird, H. W., & Gordon, E. C. (1983). *Neurological evaluation of infants and children. Clinics in Developmental Medicine, No. 84/85.* Philadelphia: Lippincott.

Ballard, J. L., Khoury, J. C., Wedig, K., Wang, L., Eilers-Waisman, B. L., & Lipp, R. (1991). New Ballard score, expanded to include extremely premature infants. *Journal of Pediatrics, 119*, 417–423.

Batchelor, E. S. (1996). Neuropsychological assessment of children. In E. S. Batchelor & R. S. Dean (Eds.), *Pediatric neuropsychology. Interfacing assessment and treatment for rehabilitation* (pp. 9–20). Boston: Allyn & Bacon.

Bayley, N. (1969). *Bayley Scale of Infant Development.* New York: The Psychological Corporation.

Blasco, P. A. (1989). Preterm birth: To correct or not to correct. *Developmental Medicine and Child Neurology, 31*, 816–826.

Bouza, H., Rutherford, M., Acolet, D., Pennock, J. M., & Dubowitz, L. M. (1994). Evolution of early hemiplegic signs in full-term infants with unilateral brain lesions in the neonatal period: A prospective study. *Neuropediatrics, 25*, 201–207.

Bradley, R. H., Whiteside, L., Mundfrom, D. J., & Blevins-Kwabe, B. (1995). Home environment and adaptive social behavior among premature, low birth weight children: Alternative models of environmental action. *Journal of Pediatric Psychology, 20*, 347–362.

Brazelton, T. B. (1973). *Neonatal Behavioral Assessment Scale. Clinics in Developmental Medicine. No. 50.* Philadelphia: Lippincott.

Brazy, J. E., Eckerman, C. O., Oehler, J. M., Goldstein, R. F., & O'Rand, A. M. (1991). Nursery Neurobiologic Risk Score: Important factors in predicting outcome in very low birth weight infants. *Journal of Pediatrics, 118*, 783–792.

Campbell, S. K., Kolobe, T. H. A., Osten, E., Girolami, G. L., & Lenki, M. (1994). *Test of Infant Motor Performance.* Chicago: Department of Physical Therapy, University of Illinois.

Capone, G. T. (1996). Human brain development. In A. J. Capute & P. J. Accardo (Eds.), *Developmental disabilities in infancy and childhood. Second edition. Vol. 1, Neurodevelopmental diagnosis and treatment* (pp. 25–75). Baltimore: Paul H. Brookes.

Capute, A. J., & Accardo, P. J. (1996). A neurodevelopmental perspective on the continuum of developmental disabilities. In A. J. Capute & P. J. Accardo (Eds.), *Developmental disabilities in infancy and childhood. Second edition* (Vol. 1, pp. 1–22). Baltimore: Paul H. Brookes.

Case-Smith, J. (1996). Analysis of current motor development theory and recently published infant motor assessments. *Infants and Young Children, 9*, 29–41.

Case-Smith, J., & Bigsby, R. (1993). *Posture and Fine Motor Assessment of Infants.* Columbus: Division of Occupational Therapy, Ohio State University.

Cherny, S. S., Fulker, D. W., Emde, R. N., Robinson, J., Corley, R. P., Reznick, J. S., Plomin, R., and DeFries, J. C. (1994). A developmental-genetic analysis of continuity and change in the Bayley Mental Development Index from 14 to 24 months: The MacArthur Longitudinal Twin Study. *Psychological Science, 5*, 354–360.

Chugani, H. T. (1992). Functional brain imaging in pediatrics. *Pediatric Clinics of North America, 39*, 777–796.

Depp, R. (1995). Perinatal asphyxia: Assessing its causal role and timing. *Seminars in Pediatric Neurology, 2*, 3–36.

Diamond, G., & Cohen, H. (1992). Developmental disabilities in children with HIV infection. In A. Crocker, H. Cohen, & T. Kastner (Eds.), *HIV infection and developmental disabilities* (pp. 33–43). Baltimore: Paul H. Brookes.

Dobbing, J., & Smart, J. L. (1974). Vulnerability of developing brain and behavior. *British Medical Journal, 30*, 164–168.

Drillien, C. M. (1972). Abnormal neurologic signs in the first year of life in low birth weight infants: Possible prognostic significance. *Developmental Medicine and Child Neurology, 14*, 575–584.

Drotar, D., & Sturm, L. (1989). Training psychologists as infant specialists. *Infants and Young Children, 2*, 58–66.

Dubowitz, L., Dubowitz, V., & Goldberg, C. (1970). Clinical assessment of gestational age in the newborn infant. *Journal of Pediatrics, 77*, 1–10.

Egan, D. F., Illingworth, R. S., & MacKeith, R. C. (1976). *Developmental screening 0–5 years. Clinics in Developmental Medicine, No. 30.* Philadelphia: Lippincott.

Ellenberg, J. H., & Nelson, K. B. (1988). Cluster of perinatal events identifying infants at high risk for death or disability. *Journal of Pediatrics, 113*, 546–552.

Elliott, C. D. (1990). *Differential Ability Scales. Introductory and technical handbook.* San Antonio: The Psychological Corporation.

Escalona, S. K. (1982). Babies at double hazard: Early development of infants at biologic and social risk. *Pediatrics, 70*, 670–676.

Fagan, J. F., & Detterman, D. K. (1992). The Fagan Test of Infant Intelligence: A technical summary. *Journal of Applied Developmental Psychology, 13*, 173–193.

Fagan, J. F., & Singer, L. T. (1983). Infant recognition memory as a measure of intelligence. In L. P. Lipsitt (Ed.), *Advances in infant research* (Vol. 2, pp. 31–78). Norwood, NJ: Ablex.

Fischer, K. W., & Pipp, S. (1984). Process of cognitive development. In R. J. Sternberg (Ed.), *Mechanisms of cognitive development* (pp. 88–148). San Francisco: Freeman.

Flanagan, D. P., & Alfonso, V. C. (1995). A critical review of the technical characteristics of new and recently revised intelligence tests for preschool children. *Journal of Psychoeducational Assessment, 13*, 66–90.

Folio, M. R., & Fewell, R. R. (1983). *Peabody Developmental Motor Scales and activity cards.* Allen, TX: DLM Teaching Resources.

Freeman, J. M., & Nelson, K. B. (1988). Intrapartum asphyxia and cerebral palsy. *Pediatrics, 82*, 240–249.

Georgieff, M. K., Bernbaum, J. C., Hoffman-Williamson, M., & Daft, A. (1986). Abnormal truncal muscle tone as a useful early marker for developmental delay in low birth weight infants. *Pediatrics, 77*, 659–663.

Giedd, J. N. (1997). Normal development. In B. S. Peterson (Ed.), *Neuroimaging: Child and Adolescent Psychiatric Clinics of North America, 6*, 265–282.

Gordon, N. (1996a). Epilepsy and disorders of neuronal migration. I. Introduction. *Developmental Medicine and Child Neurology, 38*, 1053–1057.

Gordon, N. (1996b). Epilepsy and disorders of neuronal migration. II: Epilepsy as a symptom of neuronal migration defects. *Developmental Medicine and Child Neurology, 38*, 1131–1134.

Gortmaker, S. L., Walker, P. K., Weitzman, M., & Sobol, A. M. (1990). Chronic conditions, socioeconomic risks, and behavioral problems in children and adolescents. *Pediatrics, 85*, 267–276.

Greenough, W. T., & Juraska, J. M. (1986). *Developmental neuropsychobiology.* Orlando: Academic Press.

Griffiths, R. (1970). *The abilities of young children. A comprehensive system of mental measurement for the first eight years of life.* London: Child Development Research Center.

Hallett, T., & Proctor, A. (1996). Maturation of the central nervous system as related to communication and cognitive development. *Infants and Young Children, 8*, 1–15.

Harris, J. C. (1995). *Developmental neuropsychiatry* (Vol. 1). New York: Oxford University Press.

Harris, S. R. (1991). Early identification of cerebral palsy. In M. I. Gottlieb & J. E. Williams (Eds.), *Developmental-behavioral disorders: Selected topics* (Vol. 3, pp. 67–78). New York: Plenum Medical.

Havey, A. S. (1995). Functional neuroimaging with SPECT and PET in childhood developmental disabilities. *International Pediatrics, 10,* 177–187.

Hill, A., & Volpe, J. J. (1989). Perinatal asphyxia: Clinical aspects. *Clinics in Perinatology, 16,* 435–457.

Hobel, C., Gyvarinen, M., & Okada, D. (1973). Prenatal and intrapartum high-risk screening: Prediction of the high-risk neonate. *American Journal of Obstetrics and Gynecology, 117,* 1–9.

Honzik, M. P. (1988). The constancy of mental test performance during the preschool period. In C. Rovee-Collier & L. P. Lipsitt (Eds.), *Advances in infancy research* (Vol. 5, pp. xv–xxxi). Norwood, NJ: Ablex.

Howard, J., Parmelee, A., Kopp, C., & Littman, B. (1976). A neurological comparison of preterm and fullterm infants at term conceptional age. *Journal of Pediatrics, 88,* 995–1002.

Hubel, D. H., & Wiesel, T. N. (1970). The period of susceptibility to the physiological effects of unilateral eye-closure in kittens. *Journal of Physiology, 206,* 419–436.

Huisman, M., Koopmanesseboom, C., Fidler, V., Haddersalgra, M., Van der Paauw, C. G., Tuinstra, L. G., Weisglas-Kuperas, N., Sauer, P. J., & Touwen, B. C. L. (1995). Perinatal exposure to polychlorinated biphenyls and dioxins and its effect on neonatal neurological development. *Early Human Development, 41,* 111–127.

Hunt, J. V., Cooper, B. A. B., & Tooley, W. H. (1988). Very low birth weight infants at 8 and 11 years of age: Role of neonatal illness and family status. *Pediatrics, 82,* 596–603.

Hunt, H., Brodsky, N. L., Betancourt, L., Braitman, L. E., Malmud, E., & Giannetta, J. (1995). Cocaine-exposed children: Follow-up through 30 months. *Journal of Developmental and Behavioral Pediatrics, 16,* 29–35.

Hynd, G. W., & Willis, W. G. (1988). *Pediatric neuropsychology,* New York: Grune & Stratton.

Illingworth, R. S. (1990). *Basic developmental screening 0–4 years* (5th ed.). London: Blackwell.

Johnson, C. B. (1993). Developmental issues: Children infected with the human immunodeficiency virus. *Infants and Young Children, 6,* 1–10.

Johnston, M. V., Trescher, W. H., & Taylor, G. A. (1995). Hypoxic and ischemic central nervous system disorders in infants and children. *Advances in Pediatrics, 42,* 1–45.

Kaufman, A. S., & Kaufman, N. L. (1983). *Interpretive manual for the Kaufman Assessment Battery for Children.* Circle Pines, MN: American Guidance Science.

Kennard, M. A. (1940). Relation of age to motor impairment in man and subhuman primates. *Archives of Neurology and Psychiatry, 44,* 377–397.

Kennard, M. A. (1942). Cortical reorganization of motor function: Studies on series of monkeys of different ages from infancy to maturity. *Archives of Neurology and Psychiatry, 47,* 227–240.

Knobloch, H., & Pasamanick, B. (1974). *Gesell and Amatruda's developmental diagnosis* (3rd ed.). New York: Harper & Row.

Knobloch, H., Stevens, F., & Malone, A. E. (1980). *Manual of developmental diagnosis.* New York: Harper & Row.

Konishi, Y., & Prechtl, H. F. R. (1994). Finger movements and finger postures in pre-term infants are not a good indicator of brain damage. *Early Human Development, 36,* 89–100.

Korkman, M., Kirk, U., & Kemp, S. (1997). *NEPSY.* San Antonio: The Psychological Corporation.

Korner, A. F., Stevenson, D. K., Forrest, T., Constantinou, J. C., Dimiceli, S., & Brown, B. W. (1994). Preterm medical complications differentially affect neurobehavioral functions: Results from a new Neonatal Medical Index. *Infant Behavior and Development, 17,* 37–43.

Korner, A. F., & Thom, V. A. (1990). *Neurobehavioral Assessment of the Preterm Infant.* San Antonio: The Psychological Corporation.

Kurtzberg, D., Vaughan, H. G. J., Daum, C., Grellong, B. A., Albin, S., & Rottkin, L. (1979). Neurobehavioral performance of low-birthweight infants at 40 weeks conceptional age:

Comparison with normal full term infants. *Developmental Medicine and Child Neurology, 21,* 590–607.

Lecours, A. R. (1975). Myelogenetic correlates of the development of speech and language. In E. H. Lennenberg & E. Lennenberg (Eds.), *Foundations of language development: A multidisciplinary approach* (Vol. 1, pp. 121–135). New York: Academic Press.

Lems, W., Hopkins, B., & Samsom, J. F. (1993). Mental and motor development in preterm infants: The issue of corrected age. *Early Human Development, 34,* 113–123.

Lenn, N. J. (1991). Neuroplasticity: The basis for brain development, learning, and recovery from injury. *Infants and Young Children, 3,* 39–48.

Levine, M. D. (1983). The developmental assessment of the school-age child. In M. D. Levine, W. B. Carey, A. C. Crocher, & R. T. Gross (Eds.), *Developmental-behavioral pediatrics* (pp. 938–947). Philadelphia: Saunders.

Lewis, M., & Bendersky, M. (1989). Cognitive and motor differences among low birth weight infants: Impact of intraventricular hemorrhage, medical risk, and social class. *Pediatrics, 83,* 187–192.

Lezak, M. D. (1983). *Neuropsychological assessment* (2nd ed.). New York: Oxford University Press.

Littman, B., & Parmelee, A. H. (1978). Medical correlates of infant development. *Pediatrics, 61,* 470–474.

Loehlin, J. C. (1989). Partitioning environmental and genetic contributions to behavioral development. *American Psychologist, 44,* 1285–1292.

Lou, H. C., Hanson, D., Nordentoft, M., & Pryds, O. (1994). Prenatal stressors of human life affect fetal brain development. *Developmental Medicine and Child Neurology, 36,* 826–832.

Lowe, J., & Papile, L. A. (1990). Neurodevelopmental performance of very low birthweight infants with mild periventricular, intraventricular hemorrhage. Outcome at 5 to 6 years of age. *American Journal of Diseases of Children, 144,* 1242–1245.

Luria, A. R. (1973). *The working brain: An introduction to neuropsychology.* Middlesex: Penguin Press.

Lyon, G., & Gadisseux, L. (1991). Structural abnormalities of the brain in developmental disorders. In M. Rutter & P. Casaer (Eds.), *Biological risk factors for psychosocial disorders* (pp. 1–19). London: Cambridge University Press.

MacKeith, R. (1977). Preface to the second edition. In H. F. R. Prechtl, *The neurological examination of the full-term newborn infant* (2nd ed.). *Clinics in Developmental Medicine, No. 63.* Philadelphia: Lippincott.

Mayes, L. C., Granger, R. H., Bornstein, M. H., & Zuckerman, B. (1992). The problem of prenatal cocaine exposure. A rush to judgment. *Journal of the American Medical Association, 267,* 406–408.

McCarthy, D. (1972). *McCarthy Scales of Children's Abilities.* New York: The Psychological Corporation.

Milani-Comparetti, A., & Gidoni, E. A. (1967a). Pattern analysis of motor development and its disorders. *Developmental Medicine and Child Neurology, 9,* 625–630.

Milani-Comparetti, A., & Gidoni, E. A. (1967b). Positive developmental examination in normal and retarded children. *Developmental Medicine and Child Neurology, 9,* 631–636.

Miller, G., Dubowitz, L. M. S., & Palmer, P. (1984). Follow-up of pre-term infants: Is correction of the developmental quotient for prematurity helpful? *Early Human Development, 9,* 137–144.

Miller, L. (1988). *Miller Assessment for Preschoolers.* San Antonio: The Psychological Corporation.

Miller, L. (1993). *FirstSTEP: Screening Test for Evaluating Preschoolers.* San Antonio: The Psychological Corporation.

Miller, L. J., & Roid, G. H. (1994). *The T.I.M.E. Toddler and Infant Motor Evaluation.* Tucson, AZ: Therapy Skill Builders.

Mintz, M. (1996). Neurobehavioral manifestations of pediatric AIDS/HIV-1 infection. In Y. Frank (Ed.), *Pediatric behavioral neurology* (pp. 336–365). New York: CRC Press.

Molfese, D. (1992). The use of auditory evoked responses recorded from newborn infants to predict language skills. In M. G. Tramontana & S. R. Hooper (Eds.), *Advances in child neuropsychology* (Vol. 1, pp. 1–23). Berlin: Springer-Verlag.

Molfese, D. L., & Molfese, V. J. (1979). Hemisphere and stimulus differences as reflected in the cortical responses of newborn infants to speech stimuli. *Developmental Psychology, 15*, 505–511.

Molfese, D. L., & Molfese, V. J. (1986). Psychophysiological indices of early cognitive processes and their relationship to language. In J. E. Obrzut & G. W. Hynd (Eds.), *Child neuropsychology: Theory and research* (Vol. 1, pp. 95–115). Orlando: Academic Press.

Molfese, V. J. (1989). *Perinatal risk and infant development. Assessment and prediction.* New York: Guilford Press.

Molfese, V. J. (1992). Neuropsychological assessment in infancy. In I. Rapin & S. J. Segalowitz (Eds.), *Handbook of neuropsychology, Vol. 6. Child neuropsychology* (pp. 353–376). Amsterdam: Elsevier.

Mullen, E. M. (1984). *Mullen Scales of Early Learning.* Circle Pines, MN: American Guidance Service.

Mullen, E. M. (1989). *Infant Mullen Scales of Early Learning.* Circle Pines, MN: American Guidance Service.

Mutch, L., Leyland, A., & McGee, A. (1993). Patterns of neuropsychological function in a low-birth-weight population. *Developmental Medicine and Child Neurology, 35*, 943–956.

Nass, R., & Stiles, J. (1996). Neurobehavioral consequences of congenital focal lesions. In Y. Frank (Ed.), *Pediatric behavioral neurology* (pp. 150–178). New York: CRC Press.

Nickel, R. E. (1992). Disorders of main development. *Infants and Young Children, 5*, 1–11.

Papile, L. A., Burstein, J., Burnstein, R., & Koffler, H. (1978). Incidence and evolution of subependymal and intraventricular hemorrhage: A study of infants with birthweights less than 1500 gm. *Journal of Pediatrics, 92*, 529–534.

Parker, S., Greer, S., & Zuckerman, B. (1988). Double jeopardy: The impact of poverty on early child development. *Pediatric Clinics of North America, 35*, 1227–1240.

Parmelee, A. H., Michaeles, R., Kopp, C. B., & Sigman, M. (1974). *Newborn neurological examination.* Los Angeles: UCLA Infant Studies Project.

Parry, T. S. (1992). The effectiveness of early intervention: A critical review. *Journal of Paediatrics and Child Health, 28*, 343–346.

Phillips, R. B., Sharma, R., Premachandra, B. R., Vaughn, A. J., & Reyes-Lee, M. (1996). Intrauterine exposure to cocaine: Effect on neurobehavior of neonates. *Infant Behavior and Development, 19*, 71–81.

Piper, M. C., & Darrah, J. (1994). *Motor assessment of the developing infant.* Philadelphia: Saunders.

Piper, M. C., Mazur, B., Silver, K. M., & Ramsay, M. (1988). Resolution of neurological symptoms in high-risk infants during the first two years of life. *Developmental Medicine and Child Neurology, 30*, 26–35.

Powls, A., Botting, N., Cooke, R. W., & Marlow, N. (1996). Handedness in very-low-birthweight (VLBW) children at 12 years of age: Relation to perinatal and outcome variables. *Developmental Medicine and Child Neurology, 38*, 574–602.

Prechtl, H. F. R. (1968). Neurologic findings in newborn infants after pre- and perinatal complications. In J. H. P. Jonxis, H. K. Visser, & J. A. Troelstra (Eds.), *Aspects of prematurity and dysmaturity.* (pp. 303–323). Leiden: Stenfert Kroese.

Prechtl, H. F. R. (1977). *The neurological examination of the full-term newborn infant* (2nd ed.). *Clinics in Developmental Medicine, No. 63.* London: Heinemann.

Prechtl, H. F. R. (1981). Optimality: A new assessment concept. In C. Brown (Ed.), *Infants at risk: Assessment and intervention* (pp. 1–5). Skillman, NJ: Johnson & Johnson.

Prechtl, H. F. R. (1984). Continuity and change in early neural development. In H. F. R. Prechtl (Ed.), *Continuity of neural functions from prenatal to postnatal life* (pp. 1–15). London: Spastics International Medical Publications.

Prechtl, H. F. R., & Beintema, D. (1964). *The neurological examination of the full-term newborn infant. Clinics in Developmental Medicine. No. 12.* London: Spastics International Medical Publications/Heinemann.

Prechtl, H. F. R., Ferrari, F., & Cioni, G. (1993). Predictive value of general movements in asphyxiated fullterm infants. *Early Human Development, 35,* 91–120.

Risser, A. H., & Edgell, D. (1988). Neuropsychology of the developing brain. Implications for neuropsychological assessment. In M. Tramontana & S. Hooper Eds.). *Assessment issues in child neuropsychology* (pp. 41–65). New York: Plenum Press.

Robertson, C., & Finer, N. (1985). Term infants with hypoxic-ischemic encephalopathy: Outcome at 3.5 years. *Developmental Medicine and Child Neurology, 27,* 473–484.

Roid, G. H., & Miller, L. J. (1997). *Leiter International Performance Scale—Revised.* Chicago: L. J. Stoeling.

Roland, E. H., & Hill, A. (1995). Clinical aspects of perinatal hypoxic-ischemic brain injury. *Seminars in Pediatric Neurology, 2,* 57–71.

Rosenblith, J. F. (1974). Relations between neonatal behaviors and those at eight months. *Developmental Psychology, 10,* 779–792.

Rubenstein, J. L.R., Lotspeich, L., & Ciaranello, R. D. (1990). The neurobiology of developmental disorders. In B. B. Lahey & A. E. Kazdin (Eds.), *Advances in clinical child psychology* (Vol. 13). New York: Plenum Press.

Saigal, S., Rosenbaum, P., Szatmari, P., & Hoult, L. (1992). Non-right handedness among ELBW and term children at eight years in relation to cognitive function and school performance. *Developmental Medicine and Child Neurology, 34,* 425–433.

Saint-Anne Dargassies. (1977). *Neurological development in the fullterm and premature neonate.* Amsterdam: Elsevier.

Sala, D. A., & Grant, A. D. (1995). Prognosis for ambulation in cerebral palsy. *Developmental Medicine and Child Neurology, 37,* 1020–1026.

Sameroff, A. K., & Chandler, M. J. (1975). Reproductive risk and the continuum of caretaking casuality. In F. D. Horowitz (Ed.), *Review of child development research* (Vol. 4, pp. 157–243). Chicago: University of Chicago Press.

Sameroff, A. J., Seifer, R., Barocas, R., Zax, M., & Greenspan, S. (1987). Intelligence quotient scores of 4-year-old children: Social environmental risk factors. *Pediatrics, 79,* 343–349.

Sarnat, H. B., & Sarnat, M. S. (1976). Neonatal encephalopathy following fetal distress. A clinical and electroencephalographic study. *Archives of Neurology, 33,* 696–705.

Scheiner, A. P., & Sexton, M. E. (1991). Prediction of development outcome using a perinatal risk inventory. *Pediatrics, 88,* 1135–1143.

Selzer, S. C., Lindgren, S. D., & Blackman, J. A. (1992). Long-term neuropsychological outcome of high risk infants with intracranial hemorrhage. *Journal of Pediatric Psychology, 17,* 407–422.

Shonkoff, J. P. (1982). Biological and social factors contributing to mild mental retardation. In K. A. Heller, W. H. Holtzman, & S. Messick (Eds.), *Placing children in special education: A strategy for equity.* Washington, DC: National Academic Press.

Shonkoff, J. P., & Marshall, P. C. (1990). Biological basis of developmental dysfunction. In S. J. Meisels & J. P. Shonkoff (Eds.), *Handbook of early childhood intervention* (pp. 35–52). London: Cambridge University Press.

Sobkowiak, C. A. (1992). Effect of hydrocephalus on neuronal migration and maturation. *European Journal of Pediatric Surgery*, Suppl. I, 7–11.

Stoddart, C., & Knights, R. M. (1986). Neuropsychological assessment of children: Alternative approaches. In J. E. Obruzut & G. W. Hynd (Eds.), *Child neuropsychology: Vol. 2. Clinical practice* (pp. 229–240). Orlando: Academic Press.

Taylor, H. G., Schatschneider, C., & Rich, D. (1992). Sequelae of *Haemophilus Influenzae* meningitis: Implications for the study of brain disease and development. In M. G. Tramontana & S. R. Hooper (Eds.), *Advances in child neuropsychology* (Vol. 1, pp. 50–108). Berlin: Springer-Verlag.

Thelen, E. (1995). Motor development: A new synthesis. *American Psychologist, 50*, 79–95.

Thorndike, R. L., Hagen, E. P., & Sattler, J. M. (1986). *Guide for administering and scoring the fourth edition Stanford-Binet Intelligence Scale* (4th ed.). Chicago: Riverside Publishing.

Tjossem, T. (1976). *Intervention strategies for high risk infants and young children*. Baltimore: University Park Press.

Touwen, B. C. L., Huisjes, H. J., Jurgens, V. D., Zec, A. D., Bierman, M. E. C., Smrkovsky, M., & Olinga, A. A. (1980). Obstetrical condition and neonatal neurological morbidity. An analysis with the help of the optimality concept. *Early Human Development, 4*, 207–228.

Van de Bor, M., Ens-Dokkum, M., Schreuder, A. M., Veen, S., Brand, R., & Verloove-Vanhorick, S. P. (1993). Outcome of periventricular–intraventricular haemorrhage at five years of age. *Developmental and Child Neurology, 35*, 33–41.

Volpe, J. J. (1987). *Neurology of the newborn*. Philadelphia: Saunders.

Volpe, J. J. (1992). Brain injury in the premature infant—current concepts of pathogenesis and prevention. *Biology of the Neonate, 62*, 231–242.

Wechsler, D. (1989). *Manual for the Wechsler Preschool and Primary Scale of Intelligence—revised*. San Antonio: The Psychological Corporation.

Weisglas-Kuperus, N., Baerts, W., Smrkovsky, M., & Sauer, P. J. (1993). Effects of biological and social factors on the cognitive development of very low birth weight children. *Pediatrics, 92*, 658–665.

Welch, K., & Lorenzo, A. V. (1991). Pathology of hydrocephalus. In C. M. Bannister & B. Tew (Eds.), *Current concepts in spina bifida and hydrocephalus. Clinics in Developmental Medicine, 122*, 55–82.

Yakovlev, P. I., & LeCours, A. R. (1967). The myelogenetic cycles of regional maturation of the brain. In A. Minkowski (Ed.), *Regional development of the brain in early life* (pp. 3–69). Oxford: Blackwell.

Yerbi, M. S. (1988). Teratogenicity of antiepileptic drugs. In T. A. Pedley & B. S. Meldrum (Eds.), *Recent advances in epilepsy* (Vol. 4, pp. 93–107). Edinburgh: Churchill–Livingstone.

Zupan, V., Gonzalez, P., Lacaze-Masmonteil, T., Boithias, C., d'Allest, A., Dehan, M., & Gabilan, J. C. (1996). Periventricular leukomalacia: Risk factors revisited. *Developmental Medicine and Child Neurology, 38*, 1061–1067.

Index